D1785714

YOUNG PEOPLE AND HIV/AIDS
OPPORTUNITY IN CRISIS

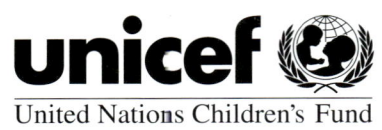 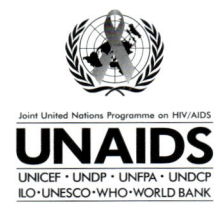 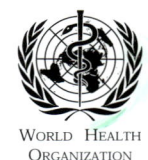

Copyright © United Nations Children's Fund, Joint United Nations Programme on HIV/AIDS
and World Health Organization, 2002

TABLE OF CONTENTS

GATESHEAD COLLEGE
Withdrawn
CENTRE 4, KNOWL...

11.8 MILLION YOUNG PEOPLE (AGED 15-24)
LIVING WITH HIV/AIDS

**7.3 million young women
and 4.5 million young men**

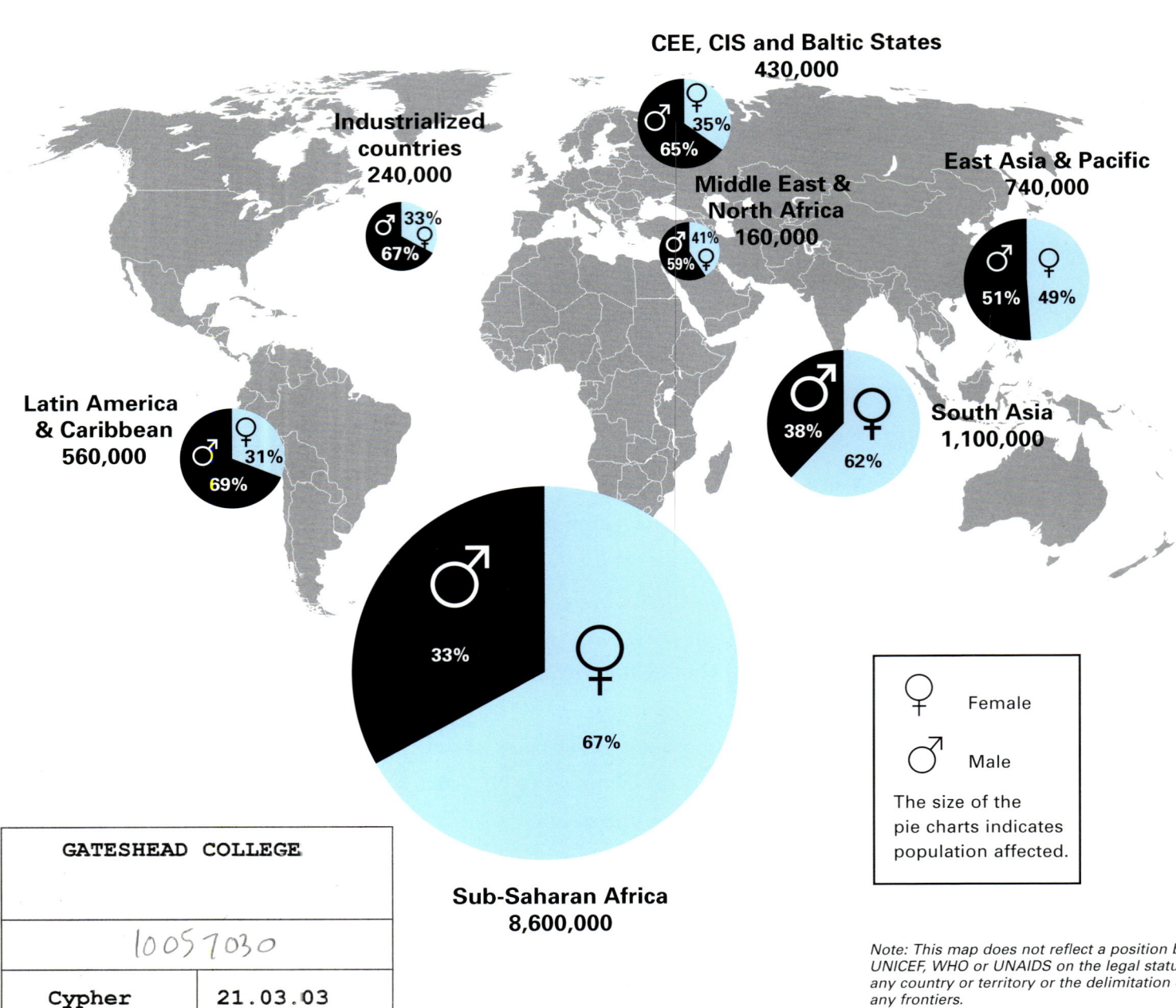

CEE, CIS and Baltic States
430,000
♂ 65% ♀ 35%

Industrialized
countries
240,000
♂ 33% ♀ 67%

Middle East &
North Africa
160,000
♂ 59% ♀ 41%

East Asia & Pacific
740,000
♂ 51% ♀ 49%

Latin America
& Caribbean
560,000
♂ 69% ♀ 31%

South Asia
1,100,000
♂ 38% ♀ 62%

Sub-Saharan Africa
8,600,000
♂ 33% ♀ 67%

♀ Female

♂ Male

The size of the
pie charts indicates
population affected.

GATESHEAD COLLEGE

10057030

Cypher	21.03.03
616.9792	£6.00
You	

Note: This map does not reflect a position by
UNICEF, WHO or UNAIDS on the legal status of
any country or territory or the delimitation of
any frontiers.

Source: UNAIDS/UNICEF, 2001.

INTRODUCTION

There is a way to halt the spread of HIV/AIDS. We must focus on young people. More than half of those newly infected with HIV today are between 15 and 24 years old.

Yet the needs of the world's 1 billion young people are routinely disregarded when strategies on HIV/AIDS are drafted, policies made and budgets allocated. This is especially tragic as young people are more likely than adults to adopt and maintain safe behaviours.

This report contains important new data about why young people are key to defeating the global HIV/AIDS epidemic, including results from more than 60 new national surveys. It reaffirms that we must accord top priority to making investments in the well-being of young people and to engaging them in the fight against HIV/AIDS.

"Global success in combating HIV/AIDS must be measured by its impact on our children and young people. Are they getting the information they need to protect themselves from HIV? Are girls being empowered to take charge of their sexuality? Are infants safe from the disease, and are children orphaned by AIDS being raised in loving, supportive environments?

"These are the hard questions we need to be asking. These are the yardsticks for measuring our leaders. We cannot let another generation be devastated by AIDS."

— Carol Bellamy
Executive Director, UNICEF

Young people are at the centre of the global HIV/AIDS pandemic. They also are the world's greatest hope in the struggle against this fatal disease.

Today's youth have inherited a lethal legacy that is killing them and their friends, their brothers and sisters, parents, teachers and role models. An estimated 11.8 million young people aged 15 to 24 are living with HIV/AIDS. Each day, nearly 6,000 young people between the ages of 15 and 24 become infected with HIV. Yet only a fraction of them know they are infected.

More than two decades into the epidemic, the vast majority of young people remain uninformed about sex and sexually transmitted infections (STIs). Although a majority have heard of AIDS, many do not know how HIV is spread and do not believe they are at risk. Those young people who do know something about HIV often do not protect themselves because they lack the skills, the support or the means to adopt safe behaviours.

Nonetheless, in areas where the spread of HIV/AIDS is subsiding or even declining, it is primarily because young men and women are being given the tools and the incentives to adopt safe behaviours. Young people have demonstrated that they are capable of making responsible choices to protect themselves when provided such support, and that they can educate and motivate others to make safe choices.

We know what works and what needs to be done.

Educating young people about HIV, and teaching them skills in negotiation, conflict resolution, critical thinking, decision-making and communication, improves their self-confidence and ability to make informed choices, such as postponing sex until they are mature enough to protect themselves from HIV, other STIs and unwanted pregnancies.

Youth-friendly services offer treatment for STIs and access to condoms and help young people become responsible for their sexual and reproductive health. Voluntary and confidential HIV counselling and testing services allow young people to determine their

HIV status and to choose safe behaviours, whether they are uninfected or infected.

We know that it is vitally important to pay special attention to vulnerable young people and those at especially high risk. We know that if HIV/AIDS prevention and care programmes are to be effective, young people must be involved in their design and implementation. We also know that keeping children in school helps protect against HIV infection.

We know that early adolescence, from the ages of 10 to 14, is a time when enduring patterns of healthy behaviour can be established, including postponing the onset of sexual activity, which can quell the spread of HIV/AIDS. Establishing healthy patterns from the start is easier than changing risky behaviours already entrenched.

"According special priority to young people will change the future course of the epidemic. Changing behaviours and expectations early results in a lifetime of benefit – both in HIV prevention and in overcoming HIV-related stigma. The challenge is to promote effective programmes that engage young people in all aspects of the response to HIV/AIDS.... In every country where HIV transmission has been reduced, it has been among young people that the most spectacular reductions have occurred."

– Peter Piot, Executive Director, UNAIDS

Parents, extended families, communities, schools and peers are critical in guiding and supporting young people to make safe choices about their health and well-being. Studies have shown that consistent, positive, emotional connections with a caring adult help young people feel safe and secure, allowing them to develop the resilency needed to manage the challenges in their lives.

No strategy to reduce the spread of HIV/AIDS can be effective unless the rights of children and young people are protected and strongly defended. No progress can be made until it becomes unacceptable to discriminate against those living with or affected by HIV/AIDS.

Communities and governments must understand the factors that increase young people's vulnerability to HIV. They must support young people with public information campaigns, both in and out of schools, to raise awareness and combat stigma. They must provide legal protection for women, people living with HIV/AIDS and children orphaned by AIDS. They also must enact and enforce legislation against the sexual exploitation of children, against early and forced marriage and against sexual violence and coercion, within and outside marriage.

All this requires strong leadership. The issues surrounding HIV/AIDS are deeply embedded in cultural and social beliefs and practices, many of them intimate, personal and private. Leadership means having the courage to meet the sexual and reproductive health needs of young people. It means working with young people to create an environment in which AIDS is not discussed in secrecy and shame, but openly and with compassion.

Leadership means making sure that every young person in every community is equipped with the facts about HIV/AIDS and how to prevent it and has access to the services, skills and support needed to develop safe behaviours from the start and to spread the message. Finally, leadership means creating a culture of zero tolerance for sexual abuse, exploitation and any form of violence against children and adolescents.

This report underscores the urgent need for governments and civil society everywhere to work with young people on effective prevention, treatment and care strategies for them. It calls for unparalleled political commitment to build the partnerships needed to raise critical financial and human resources. And it calls on adults everywhere to demonstrate their willingness to confront difficult issues.

Young people are our greatest opportunity to defeat HIV/AIDS.

Note: As a general principle, UNICEF, UNAIDS and WHO define persons between the ages of 10 and 19 as 'adolescents' and the larger age group aged 10 to 24 as 'young people'. This report uses the terms interchangeably, specifying precise age spans when appropriate.

DIFFERENT TYPES
OF AIDS EPIDEMICS
WITH YOUNG PEOPLE AT THEIR CENTRE

HIV spreads rapidly both within countries and across their borders. It affects people regardless of gender, geography or sexual orientation.

The world is now faced with a multitude of AIDS epidemics, differing in their timing, their scale and the populations they affect – and often differing even in the factors fuelling them.

In many countries the HIV epidemic is still considered 'low' or 'concentrated', confined mainly within groups at especially high risk, including males who have sex with males, people who inject drugs and those in the sex trade. An epidemic is considered 'concentrated' when less than 1 per cent of the wider population but more than 5 per cent of any 'high-risk' group are infected.

"In too many countries an official conspiracy of silence about AIDS has denied people information that could have saved their lives. We must empower young people to protect themselves through information and a supportive social environment that reduces their vulnerability to infection."

– Kofi A. Annan
Secretary-General
United Nations

In *Eastern Europe* and *Central Asia,* nearly all reported HIV infections are linked to drug injection, which has become widespread among young people, especially young men, who now make up the majority of injecting drug users. In parts of *Latin America* and *Asia* and in many *industrialized countries*, concentrated epidemics exist among men having sex with men. Several of these countries also have concentrated heterosexual epidemics among young people in the sex trade and the men who buy sex from them. In several *Middle Eastern* and *North African* countries, rates of HIV infection are rising among those who inject drugs.

In some countries of South-East Asia, such as Indonesia, Nepal and Viet Nam, epidemics are exploding among those who inject drugs and commercial sex workers, the majority of whom are under the age of 25. In China, home to a fifth of the world's people, serious concentrated epidemics have emerged in several provinces and HIV is rapidly moving into new groups.

When HIV spreads to the wider population (i.e., when more than 1 per cent of the total population is infected), the number of infections tends to rise rapidly. Such 'generalized' epidemics, found in Africa, parts of Asia, Central America and the Caribbean, account for at least four out of five new infections worldwide.

■ **Sub-Saharan Africa.** In 12 countries of sub-Saharan Africa, at least 10 per cent of those aged 15 to 49 are estimated to be infected with HIV.

The majority of new infections in this region are among young people aged 15 to 24. In Botswana, South Africa and Zimbabwe, it is estimated that more than 60 per cent of boys aged 15 today will become infected with HIV during their lifetime.

■ **Asia.** Concentrated epidemics among those who inject drugs and young commercial sex workers crossed over to the general population in Cambodia, Myanmar and Thailand, resulting in generalized epidemics in these countries. Similar patterns of transmission are being found in several southern states in India, now reporting HIV rates greater than 1 per cent among pregnant women.

■ **The Caribbean and Central America.** With 2.3 per cent of all those aged 15 to 49 infected, the Caribbean is the second-worst affected region in the world. The worst affected countries are the Bahamas, Guyana and Haiti. Most new infections are being reported among young women (aged 15-24).

■ **Eastern Europe and Central Asia.** Recent estimates of HIV prevalence in the region have found approximately 1 million persons aged 15 to 49 to be infected. This rise in infection is primarily a result of the concentrated HIV epidemic among addicted injecting drug users spreading rapidly to a wider population of occasional drug users, mostly young people, and their sexual partners.

Disadvantaged and ostracized people and communities, including people who inject drugs, those involved in the sex trade, children living on the street, school drop-outs, children orphaned by AIDS, vulnerable minorities, men who have sex with men, and children affected by armed conflict, must be urgently reached in order to protect them from getting infected and to prevent the spread of HIV to the wider population.

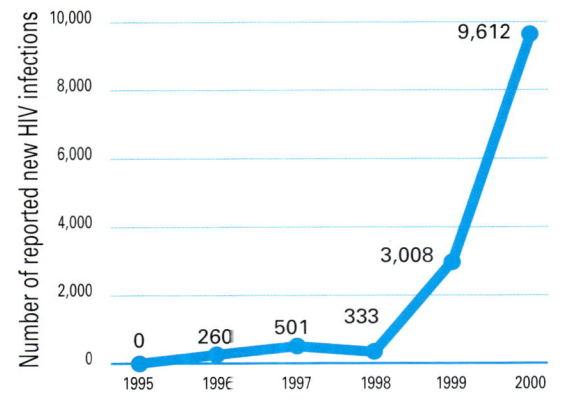

HIV EXPLODING AS INJECTING DRUG USE RISES AMONG ADOLESCENTS IN RUSSIAN FEDERATION

Reported number of new HIV infections among adolescents (aged 10-19) who inject drugs, 1995-2000

Source: European Centre for the Epidemiological Monitoring of AIDS, HIV/AIDS Surveillance in Europe, 2001.

WHY FOCUS
ON YOUNG PEOPLE?

Young people have sex

Sexual activity begins in adolescence for the majority of people. In many countries, unmarried girls and boys are sexually active before the age of 15. Recent surveys of boys aged 15 to 19 in Brazil, Hungary and Kenya, for example, found that more than a quarter reported having sex before they were 15. A study in Bangladesh found that 88 per cent of unmarried urban boys and 35 per cent of unmarried urban girls had engaged in sexual activity by the time they were 18. In rural Bangladesh, those figures were 38 per cent for boys and 6 per cent for girls.

"Young people need adult assistance to deal with the thoughts, feelings and experiences that accompany physical maturity....Evidence from around the world has clearly shown that providing information and building skills on human sexuality and human relationships help to avert health problems and create more mature and responsible attitudes."

– Dr. Gro Harlem Brundtland
Director-General
World Health Organization

Early marriage occurs across the globe, but it is most common in parts of Africa and South Asia. In Niger, 76 per cent of girls are married by 18, and in India, 50 per cent. In Nepal, 19 per cent of girls are married before they are 15 years old and 60 per cent by the time they are 18.

Adolescents who start having sex early are more likely to have sex with high-risk partners or multiple partners, and are less likely to use condoms. Delaying the age at which young people first have sex can significantly protect them from infection.

Lacking the necessary knowledge and skills, younger adolescents are less likely to protect themselves from HIV than young people in their early 20s. In Burkina

MANY HAVE SEX BEFORE THEIR 15TH BIRTHDAY

% of young men and women (aged 15-19) who had sex before age 15, 1998-2001

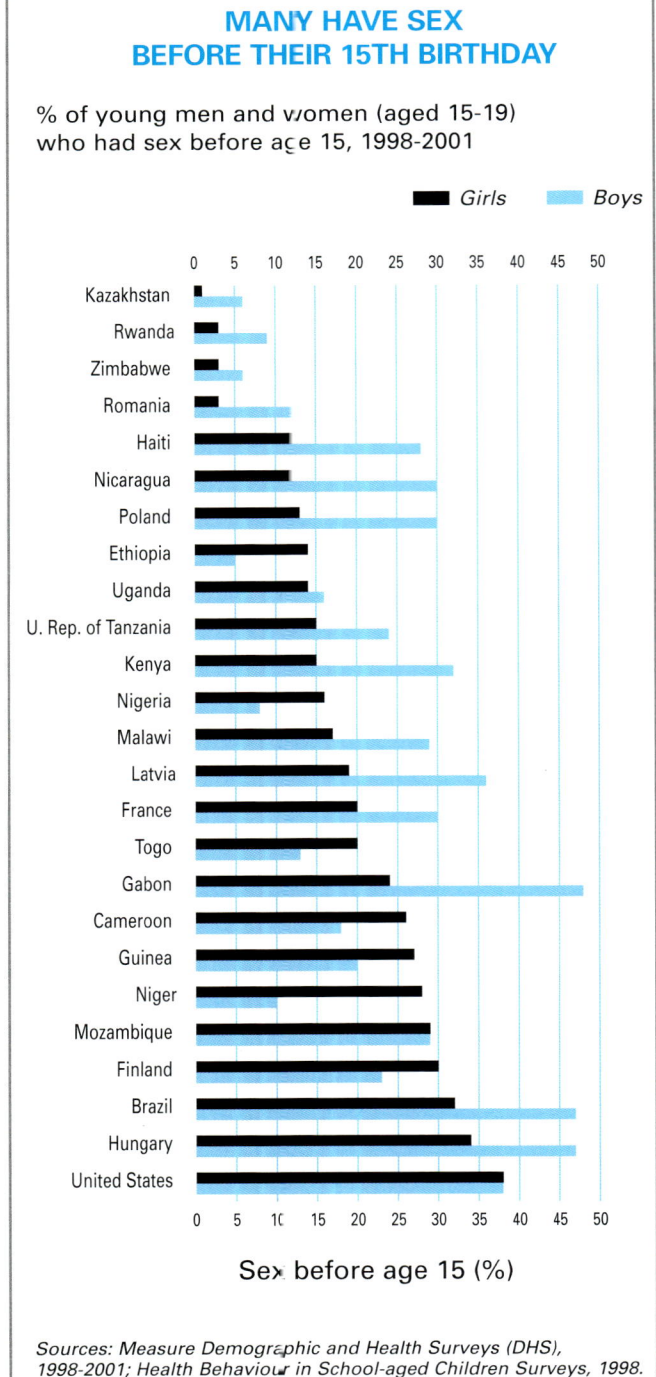

Sex before age 15 (%)

Sources: Measure Demographic and Health Surveys (DHS), 1998-2001; Health Behaviour in School-aged Children Surveys, 1998.

YOUNGER MEN LESS LIKELY TO USE CONDOMS

% of men in four sub-Saharan African countries using a condom with last non-marital, non-cohabiting partner, 1999-2001

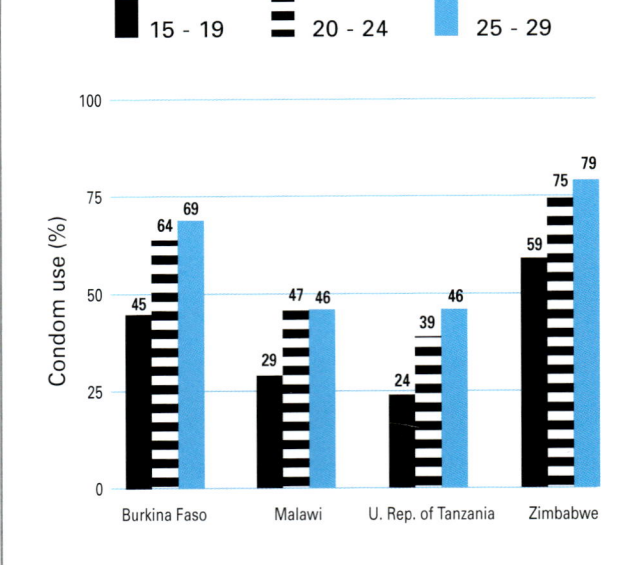

Source: Measure DHS, 1999-2001.

YOUNGER ADOLESCENTS LESS LIKELY TO USE CONDOMS AT SEXUAL INITIATION

% of adolescent girls in KwaZulu Natal, South Africa, who report a condom being used at first sexual inter-course, by age at sexual initiation, 1999

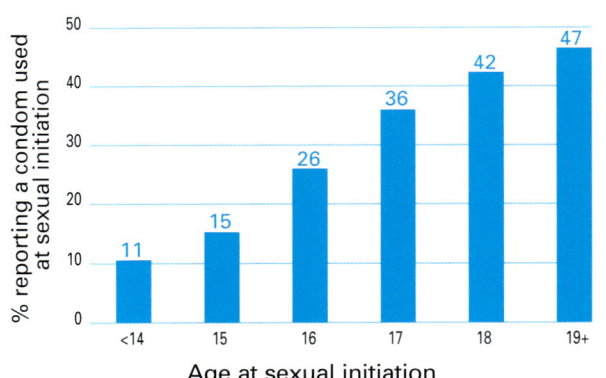

Age at sexual initiation

Source: 'Sexual initiation and childbearing among adolescent girls in KwaZulu Natal, South Africa'. Manzini, Ntsiki. Reproductive Health Matters, 9 (17): May 2001.

Faso, only 45 per cent of boys aged 15 to 19 reported using a condom with a non-marital partner, compared to 64 per cent of young men aged 20 to 24. In Malawi, 29 per cent of boys aged 15 to 19 used a condom, compared to 47 per cent of the men aged 20 to 24. In Romania, 70 per cent of boys aged 15 to 19 reported having premarital sex but only 39 per cent had used a condom their first time; 41 per cent of girls reported premarital sex but only 26 per cent had used a condom their first time. Another survey in Ukraine found that just 28 per cent of young women aged 15 to 24 had used a condom at first sexual intercourse.

Young people lack information

New studies from across the globe have established that the vast majority of young people have no idea how HIV/AIDS is transmitted or how to protect themselves from the disease.

In countries with generalized HIV epidemics, such as Cameroon, Central African Republic, Equatorial Guinea, Lesotho and Sierra Leone, more than 80 per cent of young women aged 15 to 24 do not have sufficient knowledge about HIV.

In Somalia, only 26 per cent of girls have heard of AIDS; only 1 per cent know how to avoid infection. In Ukraine, although 99 per cent of girls had heard of AIDS, only 9 per cent could correctly identify the three primary ways of avoiding sexual transmission (*see box, above*).

Two thirds of young people in their last year of primary school in Botswana thought they could tell if someone was infected with HIV by looking at them. By secondary school, a fifth of the

---

THE ABCs OF PREVENTION

Young people must be encouraged to delay sexual activity. When they become sexually active, they must be given the tools to practice safer sex.

A

Abstain from sex/delay the first sexual experience

B

Be faithful to one partner·

C

Consistently use a latex condom properly.

---

pupils still believed they could screen out risky partners by looks alone. This misinformation is especially dangerous in a country where one in three of their potential sex partners is infected with HIV.

Misconceptions about HIV/AIDS are widespread among young people. They vary from one culture to another, and particular rumours gain currency in some populations both on how HIV is spread (by mosquito bites or witchcraft, for example) and on how it can be avoided (by eating a certain fish, for example, or having sex with a virgin). Surveys from 40 countries indicate that more than 50 per cent of young people aged 15 to 24 harbour serious misconceptions about how HIV/AIDS is transmitted.

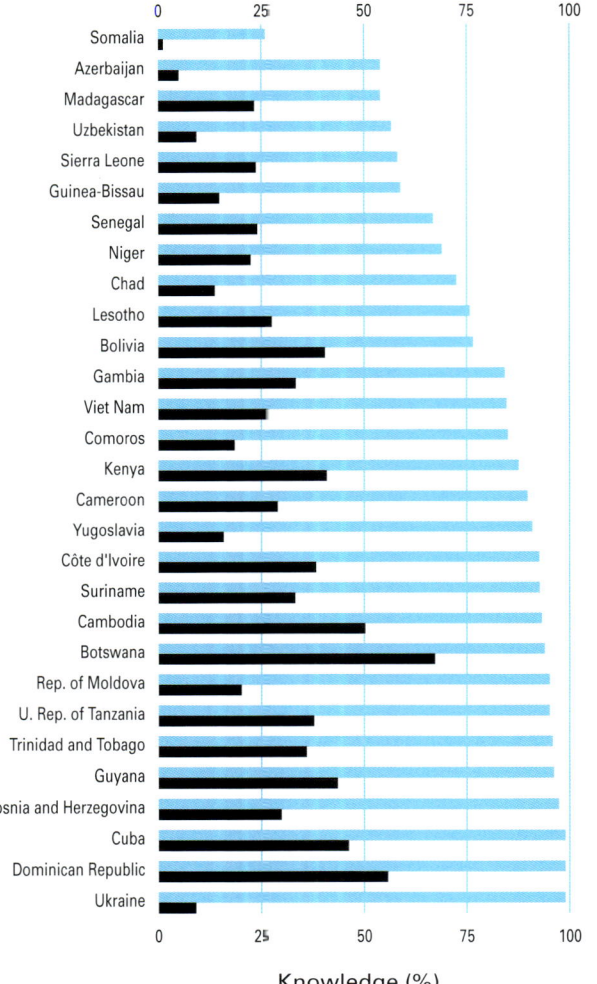

MOST KNOW LITTLE ABOUT HIV PREVENTION

% of young women (aged 15-19) who have heard of AIDS and % who know the three primary ways of avoiding infection,* 1999-2001

■ Heard of AIDS
■ Know the three main ways of protection

Somalia
Azerbaijan
Madagascar
Uzbekistan
Sierra Leone
Guinea-Bissau
Senegal
Niger
Chad
Lesotho
Bolivia
Gambia
Viet Nam
Comoros
Kenya
Cameroon
Yugoslavia
Côte d'Ivoire
Suriname
Cambodia
Botswana
Rep. of Moldova
U. Rep. of Tanzania
Trinidad and Tobago
Guyana
Bosnia and Herzegovina
Cuba
Dominican Republic
Ukraine

Knowledge (%)

*Three primary ways (ABCs):
Abstinence; **B**e faithful; **C**onsistent condom use.

Sources: UNICEF/Multiple Indicator Cluster Surveys (MICS), Measure DHS, 1999-2001.

Adolescents who are not yet sexually active must be encouraged to delay sexual activity. When young people do have sex, they must be able to protect themselves. Good-quality condoms have to be easily available and free or affordable. In some instances, however, knowledge about where to get a condom has declined. In Zimbabwe in 1999, for example, just 68 per cent of boys aged 15 to 19 knew of a specific source for condoms, compared to 77 per cent in 1994. This illustrates how vital it is to provide basic information continuously to each new group of adolescents.

Even when they do have information, some adolescents engage in unprotected sex because they lack the skills to negotiate abstinence or condom use. They may be fearful or embarrassed to talk with their partner about sex.

Still others may not adopt safe behaviours because they perceive their individual risk to be low. In Nigeria, 95 per cent of girls aged 15 to 19 perceived their risk of getting AIDS to be minimal or non-existent; in Haiti, that figure for all adolescents runs as high as 93 per cent. A study in Malawi found that girls perceived little risk in having sexual relations with a boy whose mother knew their family.

Adolescence is often a time of experimentation with drugs and alcohol. In the United Republic of Tanzania, young people aged 16 to 24 who smoke and drink alcohol are four times more likely than their peers to have multiple sex partners. In the United States of America, college students who have sex under the influence of drugs or alcohol are 2.5 times more likely not to use protection. In Buenos Aires, Argentina, a fifth of drug injectors said they started injecting when they were 16 or younger, and two thirds had started by the time they were 18.

Studies have repeatedly identified 'protective factors' that help adolescents reduce high-risk behaviours such as engaging in unprotected sex and using drugs. One recent study in rural Zimbabwe, for example, showed that being a member of a well-run community youth group reduces a young woman's risk of contracting HIV.

Protective factors include:

- Positive relationships with parents, teachers and other adults in the community

- Feeling valued

- Positive school environments

- Exposure to positive values, rules and expectations

- Having spiritual beliefs

- A sense of hope for the future.

"Boys are crying out to be heard! Most teenage boys get information concerning sex from their friends or pornographic films and literature. Some don't speak to anyone at all, and are not told anything. Those that do speak, especially to adults, are often ignored or told to 'act like a man' without being told what it is to be a man."

– Kunle Onasanya, Nigeria

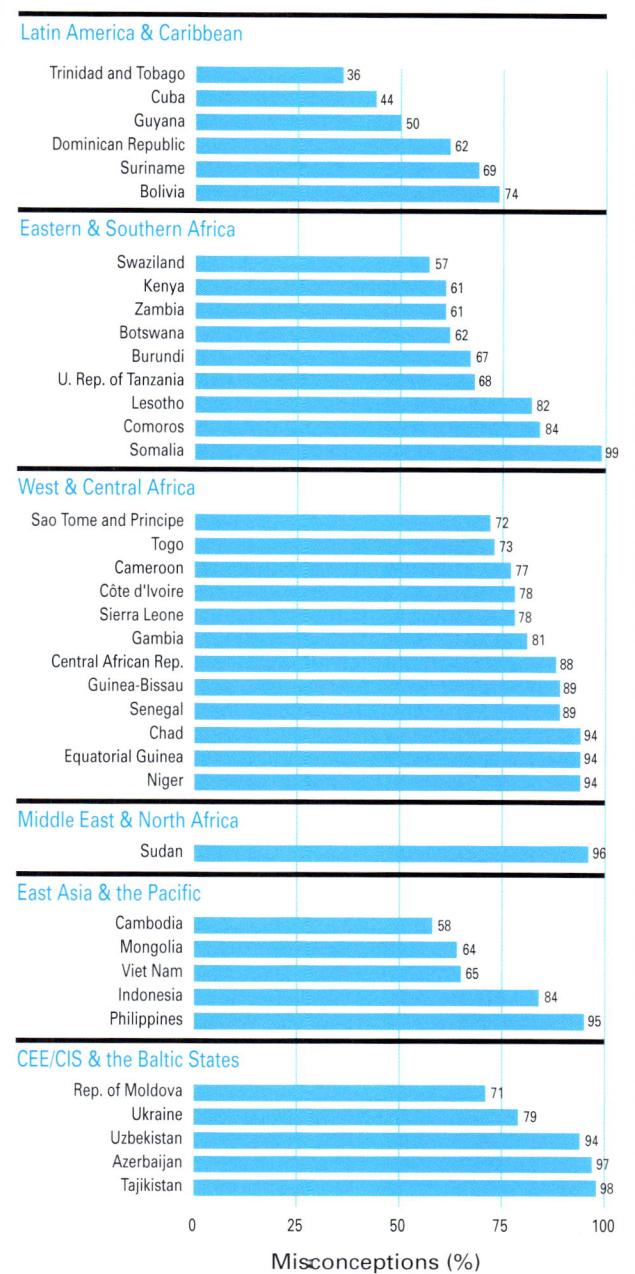

MOST GIRLS HAVE SERIOUS MISCONCEPTIONS ABOUT HIV/AIDS

% of girls (aged 15-19) who have at least one major misconception about HIV/AIDS or have never heard of AIDS, 1999-2001

Latin America & Caribbean

Trinidad and Tobago	36
Cuba	44
Guyana	50
Dominican Republic	62
Suriname	69
Bolivia	74

Eastern & Southern Africa

Swaziland	57
Kenya	61
Zambia	61
Botswana	62
Burundi	67
U. Rep. of Tanzania	68
Lesotho	82
Comoros	84
Somalia	99

West & Central Africa

Sao Tome and Principe	72
Togo	73
Cameroon	77
Côte d'Ivoire	78
Sierra Leone	78
Gambia	81
Central African Rep.	88
Guinea-Bissau	89
Senegal	89
Chad	94
Equatorial Guinea	94
Niger	94

Middle East & North Africa

Sudan	96

East Asia & the Pacific

Cambodia	58
Mongolia	64
Viet Nam	65
Indonesia	84
Philippines	95

CEE/CIS & the Baltic States

Rep. of Moldova	71
Ukraine	79
Uzbekistan	94
Azerbaijan	97
Tajikistan	98

Misconceptions (%)

Misconceptions: HIV can be transmitted through witchcraft; mosquito bites; a healthy-looking person cannot have the AIDS virus.

Sources: UNICEF/MICS, Measure DHS, 1999-2001.

TREAT STIs

Over 100 million new sexually transmitted infections (STIs), excluding HIV, occur each year among young people under 25 years of age. STIs greatly facilitate HIV transmission between sexual partners, so treating and preventing them is an important step in breaking the HIV/AIDS chain of infection. STIs that cause genital ulcers increase the risk of transmission the most. A study in South Africa showed that men infected with HSV-2 (herpes simplex virus – type 2) were seven times more likely to be also HIV positive than sexually active men who did not have HSV-2. Another landmark study in Mwanza, United Republic of Tanzania, showed that HIV incidence was 40 per cent lower after two years in communities where symptomatic STIs were better managed than in communities lacking good STI care.

STIs spread rapidly in great part because the majority of infections either do not produce any symptoms or signs, especially in females, or produce symptoms so mild that they are often disregarded. Some STI symptoms may even disappear over time, creating the false impression that the disease, too, has disappeared. Finally, many adolescents do not know the difference between normal and abnormal conditions and therefore do not know when to seek medical care.

Even when they suspect they have an infection, many young people do not seek medical care because they fear that their privacy will not be respected. They may be too embarrassed or feel too guilty to seek treatment. Services may also be inaccessible because clinics are far away or have limited hours. Health providers may be reluctant to serve adolescents. When services are located in maternal and child health centres, they are unlikely to be used by young men.

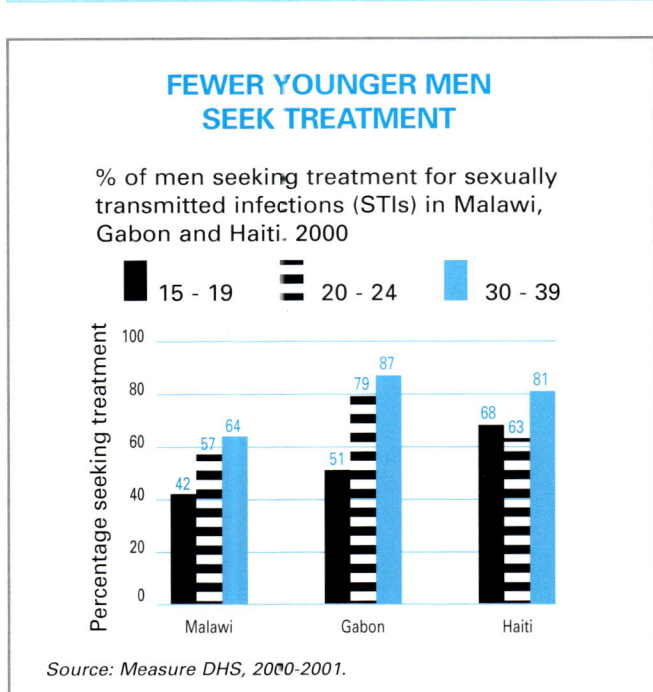

FEWER YOUNGER MEN SEEK TREATMENT

% of men seeking treatment for sexually transmitted infections (STIs) in Malawi, Gabon and Haiti, 2000

Source: Measure DHS, 2000-2001.

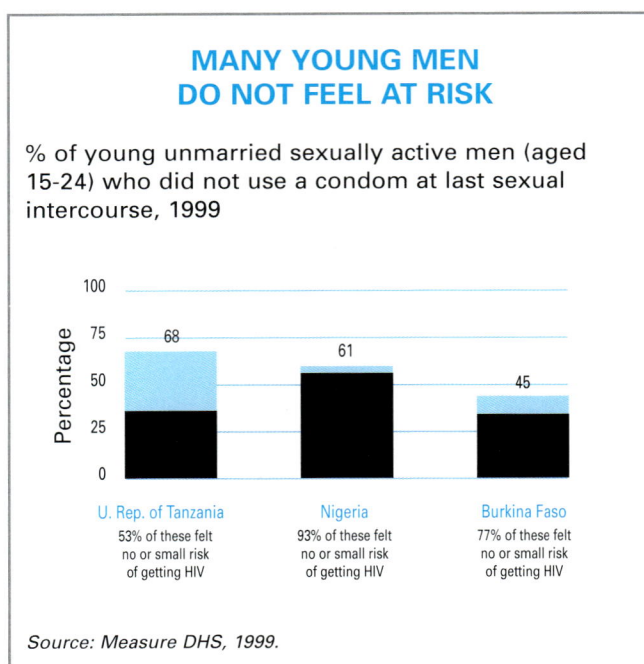

MANY YOUNG MEN DO NOT FEEL AT RISK

% of young unmarried sexually active men (aged 15-24) who did not use a condom at last sexual intercourse, 1999

Source: Measure DHS, 1999.

Girls are very vulnerable

Though as a global average there are slightly more men infected with HIV than women, adolescent girls are at very high risk of getting infected. This pattern is especially clear in sub-Saharan Africa, the region most severely affected by HIV/AIDS. More than two thirds of newly infected 15- to 19-year-olds in this region are female. In Ethiopia, Malawi, United Republic of Tanzania, Zambia and Zimbabwe, for every 15- to 19-year-old boy who is infected, there are five to six girls infected in the same age group.

There are a number of reasons why girls in sub-Saharan Africa are becoming infected younger and dying earlier than boys are. In major urban areas of eastern and southern Africa, epidemiological studies have shown that 17 to 22 per cent of girls aged 15 to 19 are already HIV infected compared with 3 to 7 per cent of boys of similar age. This indicates a 'sexual mixing' pattern whereby older men are having sex with young girls. In many countries where economic conditions make it difficult for girls to afford school fees, some seek favours of a 'sugar daddy' (an older man who offers compensation in cash or kind in exchange for sexual favours), engage in transactional sex (that is, exchange sex for money or goods on an occasional basis) or enter sex work (willingly or forced) to pay for school, support their families or take care of themselves.

This 'age-mixing' is fuelled by the dangerous myth among men in some places that having sex with a virgin can 'cure' HIV. Many men also assume that younger girls are not yet infected. Cultural norms related to sexuality prevent many girls from taking active steps to protect themselves. In cultures where it is vital for girls to be virgins at marriage, some girls protect their virginity by engaging in unsafe sexual practices such as unprotected anal intercourse.

GIRLS' VULNERABILITY

Many girls (aged 15-19) report that they were unwilling or coerced at sexual initiation. Adolescent girls in KwaZulu Natal, South Africa (1999) and Jamaica (2001)

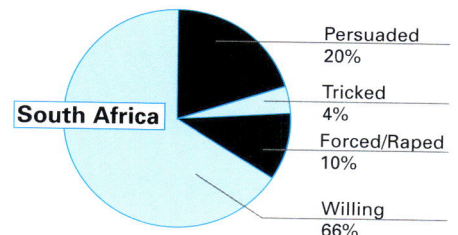

South Africa
Persuaded 20%
Tricked 4%
Forced/Raped 10%
Willing 66%

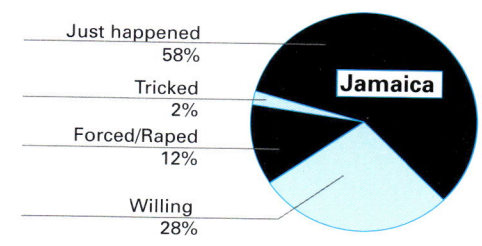

Just happened 58%
Tricked 2%
Forced/Raped 12%
Willing 28%
Jamaica

Sources: 'Sexual initiation and childbearing among adolescent girls in KwaZulu Natal, South Africa'. Manzini, Ntsiki. Reproductive Health Matters, 9 (17), May 2001; Report of Adolescent Condom Survey, Jamaica, 2001, Commercial Market Strategies / Jamaica, August 2001.

INSUFFICIENT KNOWLEDGE

% of girls (aged 15-19) who know a healthy-looking person can have the AIDS virus, 1996-2001

☐ No data ☐ 50% – 74%
■ Less than 50% ▨ 75% and over

In sub-Saharan Africa, large-scale national and regional efforts must take place in order to ensure that 90% of 15- to 24-year-olds are equipped with the knowledge and skills to protect themselves from HIV – a goal set for 2005 by the United Nations General Assembly Special Session on HIV/AIDS.

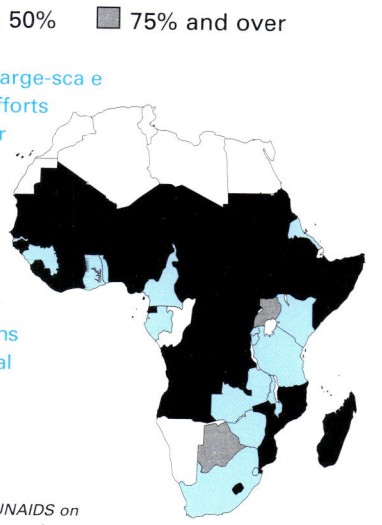

Source: UNICEF/MICS, Measure DHS,1996-2001.

Note: This map does not reflect a position by UNICEF, WHO or UNAIDS on the legal status of any country or territory or the delimitation of any frontiers.

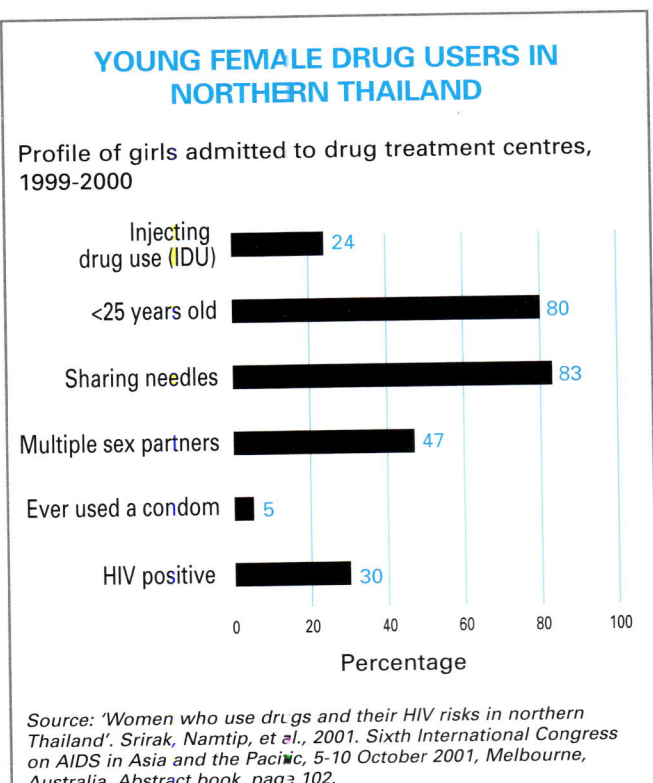

YOUNG FEMALE DRUG USERS IN NORTHERN THAILAND

Profile of girls admitted to drug treatment centres, 1999-2000

Category	Percentage
Injecting drug use (IDU)	24
<25 years old	80
Sharing needles	83
Multiple sex partners	47
Ever used a condom	5
HIV positive	30

Percentage

Source: 'Women who use drugs and their HIV risks in northern Thailand'. Srirak, Namtip, et al., 2001. Sixth International Congress on AIDS in Asia and the Pacific, 5-10 October 2001, Melbourne, Australia, Abstract book, page 102.

Biological factors also play an important role. The risk of getting infected during unprotected vaginal intercourse is always greater for women than men; and the risk for girls is further heightened because their vaginal tracts are immature and the tissues tear easily. In Kisumu, Kenya, where over a quarter of girls said that they had had sex before age 15, one in 12 contracted the virus before her 15th birthday.

The danger of infection is highest among the poorest and least powerful. Young girls living in poverty are often enticed or coerced into having sex with someone older, wealthier or in a position of authority, such as an employer, schoolteacher or older 'sugar daddy', in order to stay in school or support themselves and their families. A study in Botswana found about one in five out-of-school adolescent girls reporting that it is difficult to refuse sex when money and gifts are offered; girls as young as 13 had engaged in sex with 'sugar daddies'.

Marriage on its own offers no protection against HIV for young women, especially if their husband is much older. Another study in Kisumu, Kenya, reported that as many as half of the women with husbands at least a decade older were infected with HIV; by contrast, no women were infected whose husbands were only three years older or less. Another study of nearly 400 women attending the city's STI clinic in Pune, India, found 25 per cent infected with STIs and 14 per cent positive for HIV; 93 per cent of these women were married, and 91 per cent had never had sex with anyone but their husbands. Lacking the power to negotiate safe sex practices, many young brides may be even more vulnerable to HIV/AIDS and STIs than unmarried girls.

Interventions to stem HIV must target boys as well as girls. A mutually respectful relationship can free both young men and young women from the dangers of coerced or unwanted sex and enable them to feel comfortable discussing sexual matters and negotiating safety and protection.

Many young people are at especially high risk

Those young people who are forced to live on the social and economic margins of society have even less access to information, skills, services and support than young people normally do. If they are already living with HIV, they suffer even worse stigma and discrimination and have virtually no access to care or drugs when they fall ill.

Young people who inject drugs

Injecting drug use (IDU) is one of the many addictions that often begin during adolescence. IDU among young people, especially young men, has increased dramatically in recent years. There are more and more 'occasional' injectors, and experimentation is frequent and widespread among young people, most of whom do not consider themselves to be regular users of injecting drugs.

People who share needles and syringes for injecting drugs are at very high risk of contracting HIV. In Nepal, HIV prevalence soared among people who inject drugs from 2 per cent in 1995 to nearly 50 per cent in 1998. Half of the country's 50,000 people injecting drugs were 16 to 25 years old. A survey of addiction treatment services in Dublin, Ireland, found that 70 per cent of young people injecting drugs shared syringes.

In countries across central Asia, the Russian Federation and central and eastern Europe, it is estimated that 70 per cent of people injecting drugs are under 25 years of age. The HIV epidemic there is the world's fastest growing epidemic.

Drug dependency increases the likelihood that young people will turn to crime or prostitution to finance their drug habit. When one mixes IDU with prostitution, there is a good chance that the virus will begin to spread from those who inject drugs and their sexual partners to the wider population.

Adolescents who are sexually violated

Reported rape is on the rise in many countries, but most sexual violence still goes unreported. Both boys and girls are vulnerable to sexual violence, including abuse and exploitation, but greater numbers of girls and young women are

PROTECTING DRUG USERS IN VIET NAM

Two containers, one offering sterile needles and syringes and the other for disposal of used ones, sit in front of Hy Vong (hope) Café in Ho Chi Minh City, a needle-exchange café in Viet Nam.

Started by Save the Children Fund and supported by the Governments of Canada and Viet Nam, the café educates young people who inject drugs about the risks of HIV infection as well as providing sterile equipment. Run by the city's AIDS Committee, the café is set in a park enclosed by a wire fence. Its visitors have access to condoms, an STI clinic, hot drinks and showers. Local police have agreed not to target the park or arrest those injecting drugs there. The café, open 10 hours a day every day of the week, is run by former drug users who also provide information on preventing HIV. Around 350 people a day drop into the Hy Vong Café, many of them sex workers who also inject drugs.

victimized. Abusers are unlikely to use a condom, and the cuts and tears that result from forced sex increase the likelihood of HIV infection.

In Botswana, a 1998 study found that over two fifths of all rape cases reaching the courts involved children under the age of 16; 58 per cent were between the ages of 11 and 20. In KwaZulu Natal, South Africa, 10 per cent of adolescent girls reported their first sexual experience as forced or rape. Surveys from nine Caribbean countries found that 48 per cent of adolescent girls who had had intercourse reported that their first sexual intercourse had been forced.

The perpetrators are not always strangers. Both girls and boys are at risk of being violated by relatives, family friends, employers, teachers and other adults they may trust.

"As children, we have dreams. You dream of being a nurse or a teacher. No one dreams of being a sex worker."

– G., HIV-positive young woman, Philippines, sex worker at 16 and now a peer educator

Young people in the sex trade

It is estimated that about 1 million children are abducted or coerced into the sex trade each year. Because the commercial sexual exploitation of children is largely hidden, accurate data are difficult to collect. The Social Welfare Board of India has reported that roughly two out of five sex workers are children under 18, some as young as 8 or 9. In Moscow, Russian Federation, the average age for girls to enter prostitution is 16. Both genders are exploited; in a number of countries, such as Sri Lanka, the majority of child prostitutes are boys.

Clients often target younger adolescents because they believe that children do not carry HIV. Adolescents who are sexually exploited also have virtually no negotiating power to ask for safe sex from their exploiters. As many as 70 per cent of adolescent sex workers are HIV positive in Abidjan, Côte d'Ivoire, and 48 per cent in Pune, India. In Cambodia, where the majority of sex workers are young, over a quarter of sex workers aged 15 to 19 are infected with HIV. This points to the need to strengthen efforts to prevent young people from being ensnared in commercial sexual exploitation. Since girls rapidly become infected after entering prostitution, special efforts are also needed to identify and provide preventive services to new sex workers.

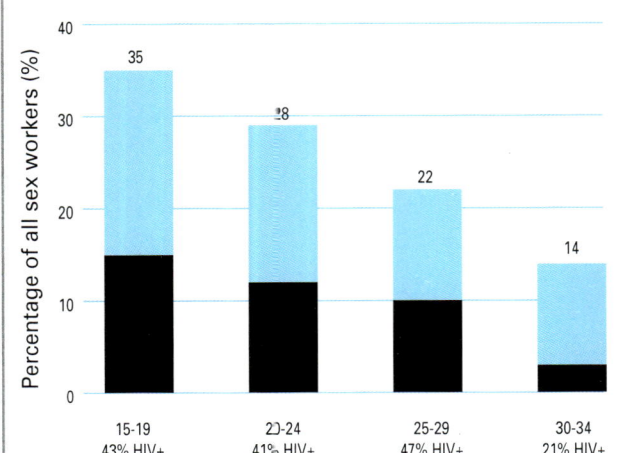

HIGH HIV PREVALENCE AMONG YOUNG SEX WORKERS

The majority of female sex workers are aged 15-24, Myanmar, 2000

Percentage of all sex workers (%)

	15-19 43% HIV+	20-24 41% HIV+	25-29 47% HIV+	30-34 21% HIV+
	35	28	22	14

Source: Sentinel surveillance data for March-April 2000, AIDS Prevention and Control Project, Department of Health, Myanmar.

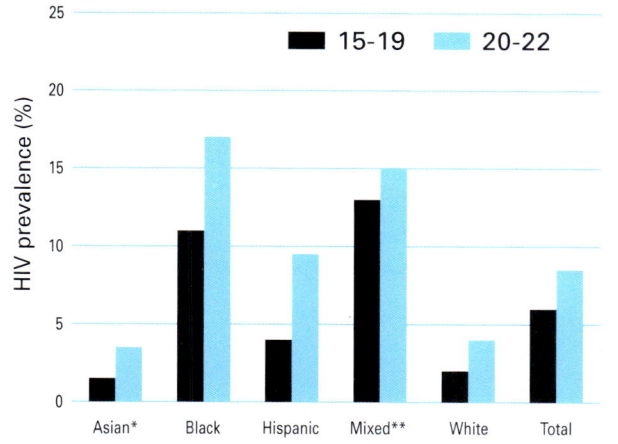

YOUNG MEN HAVING SEX WITH MEN ARE AT HIGH RISK

HIV prevalence among men who have sex with men, aged 15-22 years, by race/ethnicity and age group in select US cities, 1994-1998

Legend: ■ 15-19 ▨ 20-22

Y-axis: HIV prevalence (%)

X-axis: Asian*, Black, Hispanic, Mixed**, White, Total

*   Asian or Pacific islander.
** From multiple racial backgrounds.

Sources: 'HIV incidence among young men who have sex with men – Seven U.S. cities, 1994-2000'. McFarland, W. et al.; Morbidity and Mortality Weekly Report, 50(21), 440-4.

Children and youth on the street

Children survive on the street in every part of the world. They are the casualties of war, poverty, domestic violence, physical and mental abuse, and AIDS. Their day-to-day struggle for existence blots out any concern they might have about a disease that may kill them in the years to come.

An estimated 10,000 children live or work on the city streets of South Africa, and around 100,000 in the three Indian cities of Calcutta, Delhi and Mumbai. More than half of 141 street children interviewed in South Africa reported having exchanged sex for money, goods or protection, and several indicated they had been raped.

Young males having sex with males

The risk of contracting HIV from unprotected anal sex is especially high. The social stigma and violence visited on those identified as homosexual can magnify the risks of contracting HIV, as they may hide their sexuality and consequently do not have access to the information they need. Some young men who engage in sexual relations with other males may not identify themselves as homosexual or may have experimental and temporary homosexual experiences, without protecting themselves from unsafe behaviours that put them at risk for HIV. Among young men in Peru who identified themselves as homosexual, 40 per cent reported recent unprotected anal intercourse. In another study, over 72 per cent of young Latino men who had sex with other men in Tijuana, Mexico, and in San Diego, United States, reported unprotected anal intercourse.

Adolescents caught in armed conflict

HIV/AIDS spreads in the dislocation and destruction of armed conflict, as communities scatter and health services, educational infrastructure and legal protections collapse

At the beginning of the new millennium, 35 million people were either refugees or internally displaced, about 80 per cent of them children and women. Some young people find relative safety in refugee camps, though even there they may be victimized and abused. Many remain without any protection at all and are the targets of rape and sexual violence. They often have no access to HIV information, health care or the means to practice safer sex.

It is estimated that there are 300,000 child soldiers around the world, some as young as 10 years old. They bear arms, serve as messengers, porters or cooks, and are used for sexual services. Young men in the military tend to have multiple sex

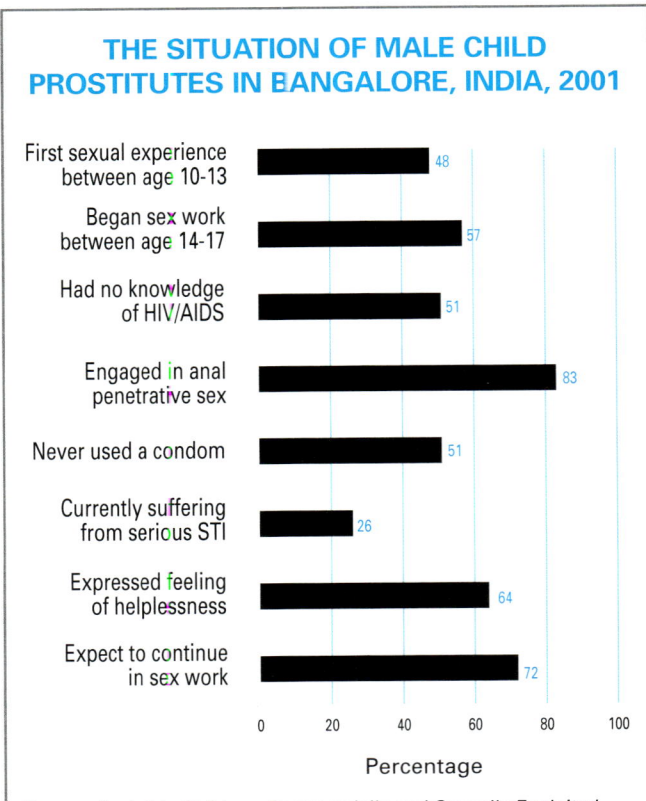

THE SITUATION OF MALE CHILD PROSTITUTES IN BANGALORE, INDIA, 2001

First sexual experience between age 10-13: 48

Began sex work between age 14-17: 57

Had no knowledge of HIV/AIDS: 51

Engaged in anal penetrative sex: 83

Never used a condom: 51

Currently suffering from serious STI: 26

Expressed feeling of helplessness: 64

Expect to continue in sex work: 72

Percentage (0, 20, 40, 60, 80, 100)

Source: 'Invisible Children: Commercially and Sexually Exploited Male Children (Male Child Prostitutes) in Bangalore, India'. Chandran, Vinay, India, 2001. Sixth International Congress on AIDS in Asia and the Pacific, 5-10 October 2001, Melbourne, Australia, Abstract book, page 21.

"Since the death of my father we have been living with our grandparents. I earn 50 or 60 rupees a day (approximately US $1.00) by selling vegetables or pulling the rickshaw. I have three younger brothers. I want to study, but my grandfather says he cannot afford to keep us in the house unless I contribute my family's share."

— 16-year-old boy orphaned by AIDS, India

partners, and military camps are often surrounded by sex workers with very high STI/HIV infection rates. Even during peacetime, young men in the military have STI rates two to five times higher than civilians – and during armed conflict, the infection rates can be 50 times higher. Often these young men return home and infect their wives or other women with HIV.

Children orphaned or affected by AIDS

Over 13 million children currently under 15 have lost one or both parents to AIDS. The total number of children orphaned by the epidemic is forecast to more than double by 2010.

Children orphaned by AIDS are at greater risk of malnutrition, illness, abuse, child labour and sexual exploitation than children orphaned by other causes, and these factors increase their vulnerability to HIV infection. They also suffer the stigma and discrimination often associated with HIV/AIDS and may be denied education, work, housing and other basic needs as a result.

Girls are likely to drop out of school to care for parents infected with HIV or for younger siblings. Orphans also leave school because of discrimination, emotional distress or because they cannot afford to pay school fees.

A study of commercial farms in Zimbabwe found that nearly half the orphans of primary school age had dropped out, and none had continued into secondary school. In Uganda, a quarter of children aged 13 to 18 whose parents have HIV/AIDS drop out of school. Children who leave school are less likely to develop the skills necessary to abstain from sex or practise safe sex; they are economically vulnerable and open to sexual exploitation.

Young people are reversing the trends

When serious and sustained efforts are made to ensure that young people live in a supportive environment and have the knowledge, skills and services to protect themselves, HIV rates decline:

■ *In Thailand,* the Government carried out a campaign promoting '100 per cent condom use' in brothels and embarked on an ambitious effort to change male attitudes towards women. Young men reduced their visits to sex workers by almost half between 1991 and 1995. Their condom use increased from 60 per cent to nearly 95 per cent. The net result was a drop in the percentage of young men infected with HIV from 8 per cent in 1992 to less than 3 per cent by 1997.

■ *In Kampala, Uganda,* HIV prevalence rates among pregnant girls aged 15 to 19 fell from 22 per cent in 1990 to 7 per cent in 2000, most likely because of delayed first intercourse, fewer partners and increased condom use. The President of Uganda has spoken openly about AIDS, and the mass media as well as the Government and community and religious organizations have active public education campaigns.

■ *In Lusaka, Zambia,* HIV prevalence among adolescents aged 15 to 19 declined from 28 per cent in 1993 to 15 per cent in 1998. There is also evidence of increased condom use and fewer sexual partners, attributed to a vigorous programme providing life skills education and health services for young people.

■ *In Brazil,* widespread information campaigns and prevention services have yielded positive results: in 1999 half the young men having sex for the first time used a condom, compared to fewer than 5 per cent in 1986, and condom sales rocketed from 70 million in 1993 to 320 million in 1999.

LEADERSHIP ON A GLOBAL SCALE

At the United Nations General Assembly Special Session on HIV/AIDS in June 2001, Heads of State and Government committed themselves to meeting a number of key goals to diminish HIV prevalence among young people aged 15 to 24. These include:

■ Reducing HIV prevalence among the young by 25 per cent in the most affected countries by 2005, and by 25 per cent worldwide by 2010.

■ Ensuring that young people have the information, education, services and life skills to reduce their vulnerability to HIV, reaching 90 per cent by 2005 and 95 per cent by 2010.

Additional goals address gender discrimination and the problems of young people who are especially vulnerable. A complete list of the goals is available at www.unaids.org, the website of the Joint United Nations Programme on HIV/AIDS (UNAIDS).

NATIONAL COMMITMENT COUNTS

Decreases in HIV prevalence among young pregnant women in Kampala, Uganda, 1990-2000

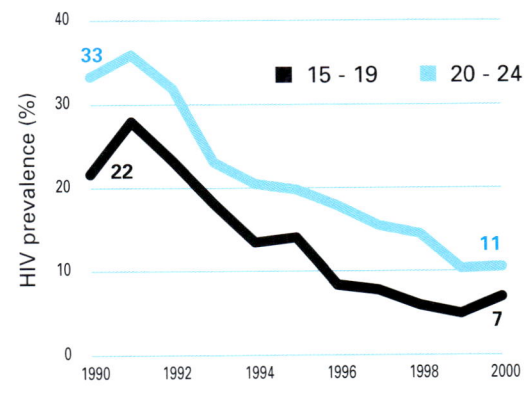

Source: National STD/AIDS Programme, Uganda, 2001.

THE WAY FORWARD

Prevention is the key to reducing infection rates and ultimately defeating AIDS. Interventions must be relevant to local conditions. And they must be tailored to the differences between boys and girls, young people living in rural and urban areas, children in school and out of school, younger and older adolescents and young people married and unmarried. Policy makers must recognize that young people, especially girls, need to have their rights protected. HIV prevention efforts must also recognize young people's immediate needs for shelter and food, as well as their need to earn an income in safe and non-exploitative ways.

Governments can contain the epidemic at relatively low cost by investing in prevention *before* HIV/AIDS becomes a significant health issue and by providing young people at especially high risk of contracting HIV with the information and support they need to prevent infection

This report advocates a ten-step strategy to prevent HIV/AIDS. The steps reinforce one another and can be adapted by countries according to their resources and the stage of their epidemics.

TEN STEPS

1 End the silence, stigma and shame.

The fear of stigma and deep-rooted discrimination makes young people less likely to adopt preventive strategies such as using condoms, seeking testing for HIV and other STIs, adhering to treatment or disclosing their HIV status to sexual partners.

National and community leadership must break the silence, challenge the stigma and eliminate the shame associated with HIV/AIDS. Presidents, prime ministers, youth leaders, entertainers, sports figures, religious leaders and other influential individuals must have the courage to talk openly and without judgement about adolescent sexuality, about violence against girls and women and about drug use. Policy makers must ensure that adolescents have the information, services and support they need. Leaders must marshal the necessary financial resources for the fight against AIDS and develop strategies based on thorough analysis of the local situation. In countries where strong political leadership has fostered openness about the issues and wide-ranging responses – examples include Brazil, Senegal, Thailand and Uganda – the tide is turning and clear successes are being achieved.

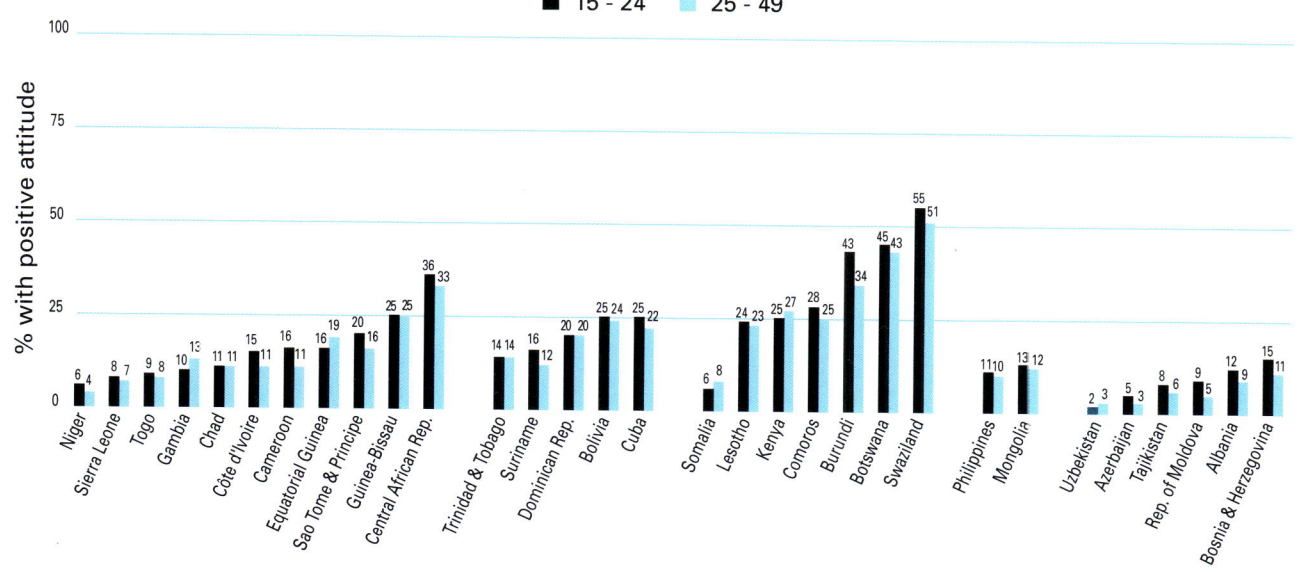

FEAR AND PREJUDICE STILL COMMON TOWARDS THOSE WITH HIV/AIDS

% of women who express a positive attitude towards people living with HIV/AIDS in response to two questions* among those who have heard of AIDS, 1999-2001

Legend: ■ 15 - 24 ■ 25 - 49

(y-axis: % with positive attitude, scale 0 to 100)

Niger 6, 4; Sierra Leone 8, 7; Togo 9, 8; Gambia 10, 13; Chad 11, 11; Côte d'Ivoire 15, 11; Cameroon 16, 11; Equatorial Guinea 19, 16; Sao Tome & Principe 20, 16; Guinea-Bissau 25, 25; Central African Rep. 36, 33; Trinidad & Tobago 14, 14; Suriname 16, 12; Dominican Rep. 20, 20; Bolivia 25, 24; Cuba 25, 22; Somalia 6, 8; Lesotho 24, 23; Kenya 25, 27; Comoros 28, 25; Burundi 43, 34; Botswana 45, 43; Swaziland 55, 51; Philippines 11, 10; Mongolia 13, 12; Uzbekistan 2, 3; Azerbaijan 5, 3; Tajikistan 8, 6; Rep. of Moldova 9, 5; Albania 12, 9; Bosnia & Herzegovina 15, 11

*1. Should a teacher who is HIV positive but looks healthy be allowed to continue working?
2. Would you buy food from an HIV-positive shopkeeper?

Source: UNICEF/MICS, 1999-2001.

2 Provide young people with knowledge and information.

Young people cannot protect themselves if they do not know the facts about HIV/AIDS. Adolescents must learn the facts *before* they become sexually active, and the information needs to be regularly reinforced and built on, both in the classroom and beyond. A basic education of good quality for all children, offering sound knowledge about sexuality and HIV, is essential.

BREAKING TABOOS IN EGYPT

In Egypt, a 20-minute television programme, *Youth Whispers,* airs once a week, encouraging young people to voice their views on issues that concern them. Featuring interviews with young people, studio discussions with them and their parents, and quiz questions, the programme offers young people important information they can use in their lives and increases community awareness about issues of concern for young people. The show is extremely popular and adolescents are actively involved in developing its content. The programme, developed by UNICEF and the Egyptian AIDS Society, has addressed such themes as attempted suicide, mother-daughter relationships, trust and confidentiality, and reproductive health.

...Increasing knowledge through schools

Many adults fear that informing young adolescents about sex and teaching them how to protect themselves will make them sexually active. In surveys from Cambodia, Haiti, Malawi and Zimbabwe, at least 40 per cent of adults felt that children aged 12 to 14 should not be taught to use condoms. But a review of more than 50 sex education programmes around the world found that young people are more likely to delay starting their sexual activity when they are provided with correct information about sexual and reproductive health. And when they do start having sex, they are more likely to protect themselves against unwanted pregnancy and STIs including HIV.

Good-quality education fosters analytical thinking and healthy habits. Better-educated young people are more likely to acquire the knowledge, confidence and social skills to protect themselves from the virus. In Zambia, where more than 20 per cent of adults are living with HIV, adolescents with more years of schooling are less likely to have casual partners and more likely to use condoms than are their peers with less schooling.

It is also essential to reach young people before they engage in high-risk behaviours, including drug and alcohol use. Information on HIV/AIDS and reproductive health, as well as life skills, should be integrated into primary school curricula and offered throughout the school years.

Starting early also means that children who do not remain in school can be reached. In India, 42 per cent of boys and 59 per cent of girls aged 15 to 17 are not in school, yet HIV/AIDS education is often introduced in schools only for children aged 15 and older. Education for HIV prevention should be timely, age-appropriate and relevant to the situations and culture of schoolchildren and their families.

...Increasing knowledge through communities

More than 120 million children of primary school age are not in school; 53 per cent of them are girls, and the gender gap widens further in secondary school. Those most likely to be out of school are children in rural, poor or isolated areas, married adolescents, working and exploited children, children affected by armed conflict and AIDS, children with disabilities and children of poor families and minorities.

In a number of African countries, AIDS has claimed the lives of such large numbers of teachers that schools have been closed and schooling has been severely disrupted. In sub-Saharan Africa, more than 40 million children of primary school age are not in school.

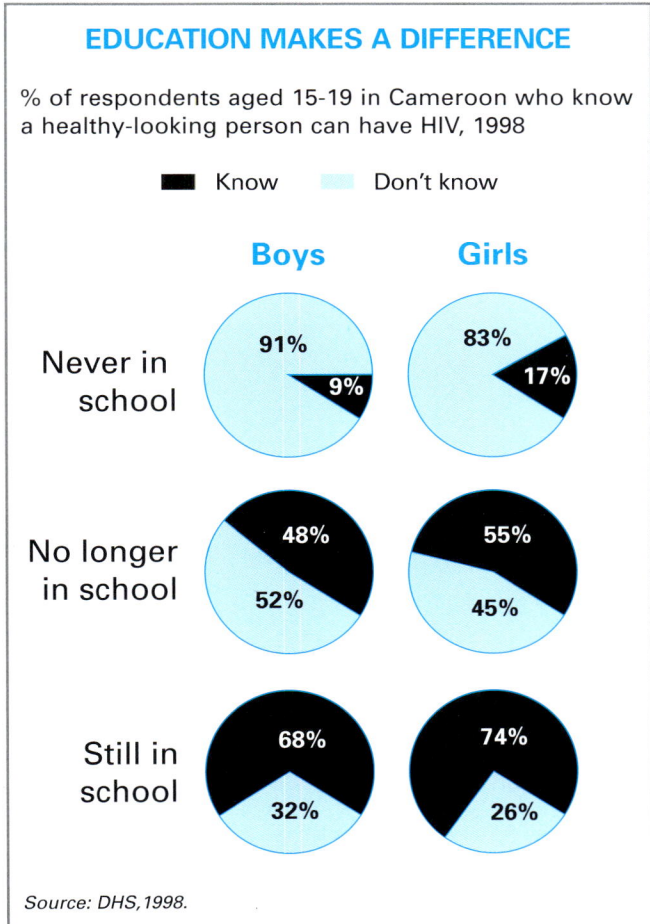

EDUCATION MAKES A DIFFERENCE

% of respondents aged 15-19 in Cameroon who know a healthy-looking person can have HIV, 1998

■ Know   ▢ Don't know

Boys   **Girls**

Never in school: 91% / 9% — 83% / 17%

No longer in school: 48% / 52% — 55% / 45%

Still in school: 68% / 32% — 74% / 26%

Source: DHS, 1998.

"Above all, we must summon the courage to talk frankly and constructively about sexuality. We must recognize the pressures on our children to have sex that is neither safe nor loving. We must provide them with information, communications skills and, yes, condoms."

– Pascoal Mocumbi, Prime Minister of Mozambique, speaking in June 2001

All sectors of society must be mobilized to reach young people out of school. Programmes that enable young people to develop a range of skills – including literacy and numeracy, and technical, entrepreneurial, practical and managerial skills – can also provide reproductive health education for the most excluded children, including young mothers at home, children living on the street and working children.

Parents and community and religious leaders need to recognize the importance of their own roles in providing life-saving information and skills. In Masaka, Uganda, health workers have taken on the role of traditional *sengas* (usually paternal aunts) who give guidance to adolescent girls. In rural Zambia, birth attendants and traditional chiefs travel in teams to deliver the facts about HIV and lift the taboo on providing sex education to young adolescents. In an AIDS prevention programme in India, *mahila mandals* or women's village councils reach out to young women.

In homes where families communicate openly about sexuality, young people often make safer choices with regard to sex. But many parents are unwilling to talk about sex or uncomfortable doing so, or they may lack the knowledge themselves. More programmes are needed that help parents and other adults in the community overcome their discomfort as well as their lack of information. A few examples:

■ In Adjumani district, northern Uganda, meetings were set up with small groups of parents to give them the knowledge and confidence to talk to their children about reproductive health. After a year, half had begun talking to their children, although 10 per cent still preferred aunts or other close relatives to provide the information and another 10 per cent preferred community health workers to do it.

■ In Kenya, religious leaders are delivering messages about HIV and AIDS to their communities. A guide was designed to improve communication between parents and children, and 5,000 copies were distributed through churches. The clergy have also used the guide to help advise parents.

■ In Chile, Mexico and Peru, school-based sexuality education programmes include special activities to involve parents – a component that has helped to convince school administrators and teachers of the value of the programme.

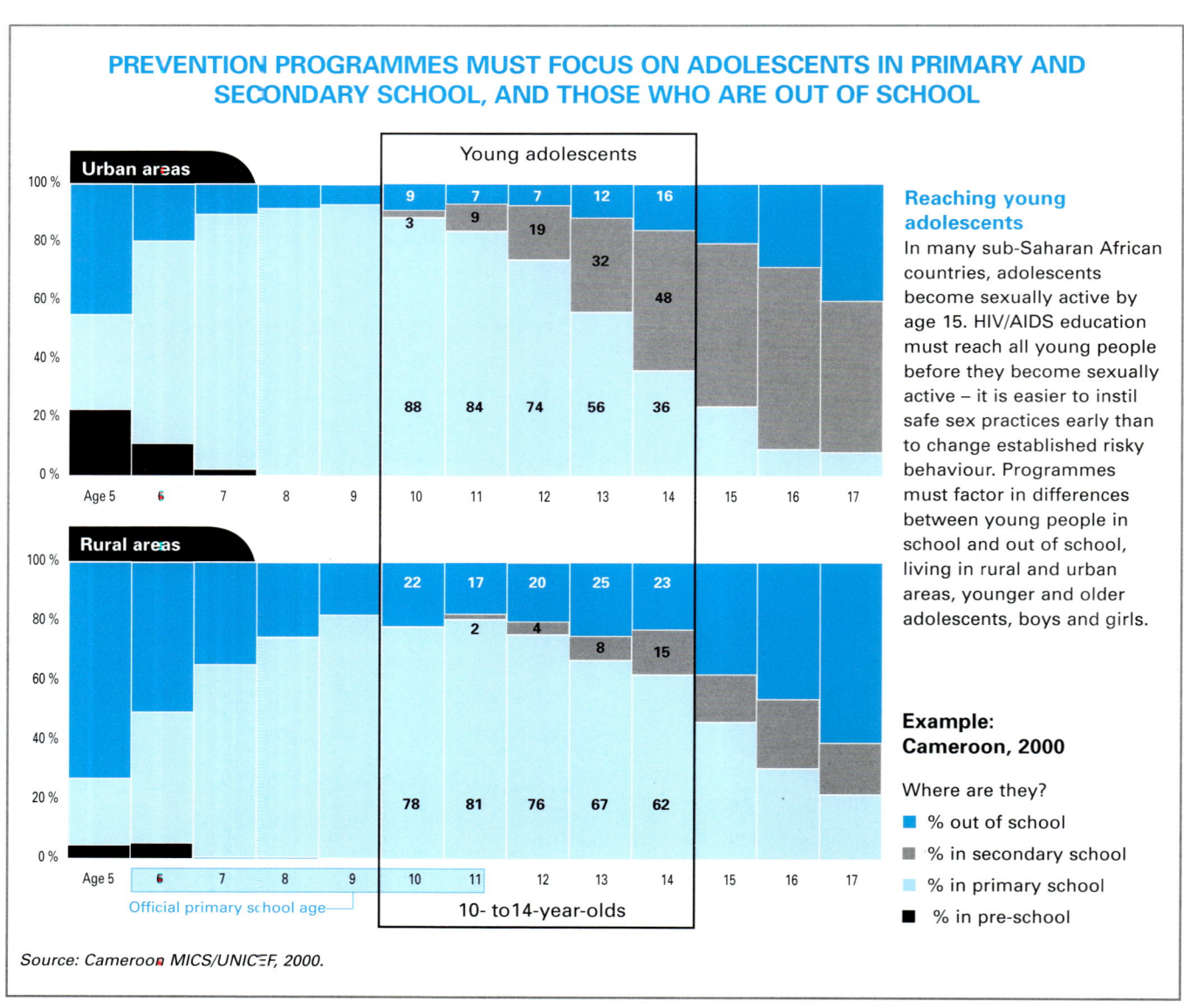

PREVENTION PROGRAMMES MUST FOCUS ON ADOLESCENTS IN PRIMARY AND SECONDARY SCHOOL, AND THOSE WHO ARE OUT OF SCHOOL

Reaching young adolescents

In many sub-Saharan African countries, adolescents become sexually active by age 15. HIV/AIDS education must reach all young people before they become sexually active – it is easier to instil safe sex practices early than to change established risky behaviour. Programmes must factor in differences between young people in school and out of school, living in rural and urban areas, younger and older adolescents, boys and girls.

Example: Cameroon, 2000

Where are they?

■ % out of school
■ % in secondary school
■ % in primary school
■ % in pre-school

Source: Cameroon MICS/UNICEF, 2000.

"We will promote effective means of [AIDS] prevention, practices that save lives, and behaviour that minimizes the risk of infection. In doing so, we will support the churches' historic commitment to faithfulness and abstinence, while recognizing that life may present us with contexts in which these ideals are unachievable."

> – Global consultation, Ecumenical Response
> to the Challenge of HIV/AIDS in Africa,
> November 2001

...Increasing knowledge through the media

The mass media are a powerful weapon against HIV/AIDS. Media campaigns that use famous actors, athletes or musicians provide role models for young people. The media can disseminate information among young people, such as the ABCs of HIV prevention *(see box on page 13)*. The media can also tackle difficult issues such as how to handle unwanted sexual advances, negotiate condom use and redefine what it means to be a 'real man'. Good programming in the mass media can counter popular misconceptions about adolescents, reveal the discrimination and abuse young people face and highlight the contributions they make to their communities.

In order to be effective, the media should involve young people at all stages to ensure that what is said will be understood, disseminated in an effective format and accessible to young people. Information should not be withheld, and facts should be presented in an honest, non-judgemental way. The greatest benefits are gained when young people have access to the health services,

condoms and other social support they need to follow through on the media messages and change their behaviour.

While the mass media provide wide outreach, different types of theatre and entertainment as well as the Internet have been used to break the silence surrounding HIV/AIDS. In Brazil, street theatre was part of a programme for young people that has been credited with increasing their condom use. A competition in Burkina Faso, Mali and Senegal asked adolescents to script a short film on HIV/AIDS and attracted many young people keen for the prize: to have their film made by one of Africa's leading directors.

In South Africa, *Soul Buddyz,* a weekly television drama, runs in tandem with a radio series, both of them focusing on issues that range from adolescent sexuality, HIV/AIDS and children's rights, to road safety, gun safety and bullying. By presenting fictional characters who make informed choices, the programmes provide positive role models for adolescents.

3 Equip young people with life skills to put knowledge into practice.

Behaviour is not changed by knowledge alone. Young people need skills to put what they learn into practice. *Life skills* – skills in negotiation, conflict resolution, critical thinking, decision-making and communication – are vital for young people. These skills help boys and girls learn to relate to one another as equals, work in groups, build self-esteem, resolve disagreements peacefully and resist both peer and adult pressure to take unnecessary risks. Life skills can be taught in many creative and innovative ways, both in and out of school.

In Namibia, young people are facilitating life skills training to reduce teenage pregnancy and prevent HIV/AIDS, substance abuse and rape. The young people who have been trained have so far reached 100,000 of their peers both in and out of school. In Bangladesh, life skills training has been linked with training to develop marketable skills and employment opportunities: 20,000 girls and young women have received non-traditional education, skills training and credit through the Bangladesh Centre of Mass Education and Science.

In Viet Nam, schoolchildren in grades 1 to 12 are using role play and other interactive methods to learn how to protect themselves from HIV/AIDS and other STIs.

Before the project began, teams of youth researchers collected data both in schools and elsewhere from children aged 10 to 18, their teachers, their parents and the broader community. These data helped to pinpoint the nature of the problems, laying the groundwork for developing the life skills programme and for monitoring progress over time.

Key elements are the training and support for teachers to introduce the new techniques. The Government has underwritten the project from the start and is fully committed to sustaining and expanding the activities.

The life skills training has been adapted for use throughout Viet Nam in a variety of settings, reaching children and adolescents living on the street as well as schoolchildren, helping them to handle their sexuality issues and protect themselves from HIV/AIDS, sexual abuse and drug abuse. By early 2000, the Ministry of Education and Training had integrated the approach in health education classes in primary schools and was expanding the life skills approach across the nation's secondary schools.

4 Provide youth-friendly health services.

Youth-friendly health services can be free-standing clinics or attached to existing clinics or recreational facilities. Ideally, they provide a full range of services and information to young people and are welcoming, confidential, conveniently located and affordable. The staff members do not patronize or lecture young people and give them plenty of time to talk.

The services to help prevent HIV and other STIs include access to condoms and voluntary counselling and testing for HIV. For young women who are pregnant and HIV positive, the clinics provide information and services to help them avoid transmitting HIV to their infants.

In Thailand, 'health corners' for adolescents have been set up in health clinics. The Self Center programme in the United States deploys teams of nurses and social workers who divide their time between schools and the clinic. The teams present classes on reproductive health, values and decision-making; run informal discussion groups about development in puberty, drug use and parenting; and provide individual counselling sessions when needed. At the clinic, the teams provide more extensive counselling on reproductive health and arrange referrals for young people requiring medical care.

In Zambia, young peer educators have teamed up with nurses in youth-friendly clinics to provide information on HIV/AIDS, other STIs and illnesses, and pregnancy, while the clinic staff provide STI treatment. The clinics issue condoms and offer counselling and support on relationships, rape and other issues. Well-regarded and respected in their communities, the peer educators also use drama, poetry, music and the electronic media to reach a wider public.

In each district a youth advisory committee, which meets monthly, serves as a link between the community and the clinic. The clinics also maintain close contact with the police, who have been trained to handle abuse cases and refer the victims for counselling and help. The clinics' staff meet monthly to discuss statistics, share experiences and collaborate on problem-solving.

Zambia's first youth-friendly clinics were established in 1996 in Lusaka, the country's capital, by the city's health board in partnership with non-governmental organizations. The lessons learned in Lusaka have since been applied elsewhere. By the end of 2001, five districts in Zambia were home to 63 youth-friendly clinics staffed by more than 200 peer educators and supported by the Government of the United Kingdom, UNICEF and other agencies.

5 Promote voluntary and confidential HIV counselling and testing.

Nine out of 10 people living with HIV/AIDS do not know they are infected. Yet studies have shown that young people have a strong interest in knowing their HIV status. More than 75 per cent of young people surveyed in Kenya, and about 90 per cent in Uganda, indicated that they would like to be tested while still healthy.

Voluntary and confidential HIV counselling and testing (VCT) is an important tool for preventing HIV. VCT allows adolescents to evaluate their behaviour and its consequences. A negative test result offers a key opportunity to reinforce the importance of safety and risk-reduction behaviours. Young people who test HIV positive must receive referrals for care and opportunities to talk to knowledgeable people who can help them understand what their HIV status means and the

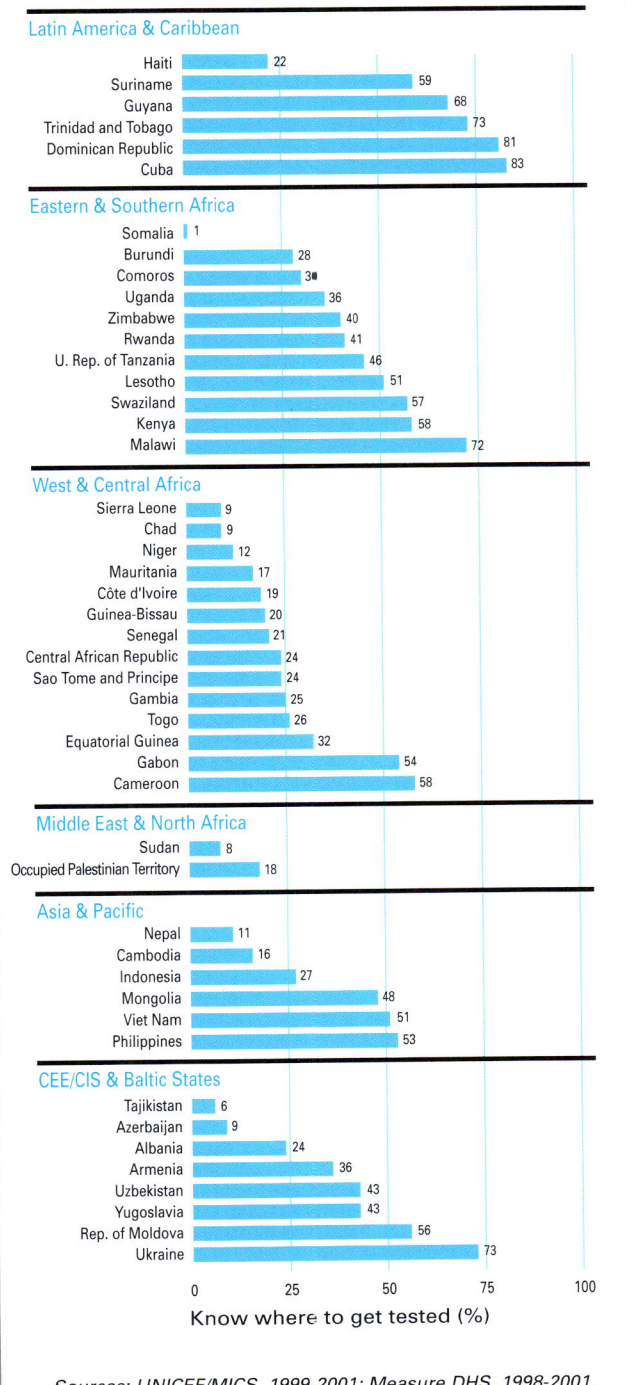

FEW YOUNG WOMEN KNOW WHERE TO GET TESTED FOR HIV

% of young women (aged 15-19) who know where to get tested, 1998-2001

Latin America & Caribbean
- Haiti: 22
- Suriname: 59
- Guyana: 68
- Trinidad and Tobago: 73
- Dominican Republic: 81
- Cuba: 83

Eastern & Southern Africa
- Somalia: 1
- Burundi: 28
- Comoros: 30
- Uganda: 36
- Zimbabwe: 40
- Rwanda: 41
- U. Rep. of Tanzania: 46
- Lesotho: 51
- Swaziland: 57
- Kenya: 58
- Malawi: 72

West & Central Africa
- Sierra Leone: 9
- Chad: 9
- Niger: 12
- Mauritania: 17
- Côte d'Ivoire: 19
- Guinea-Bissau: 20
- Senegal: 21
- Central African Republic: 24
- Sao Tome and Principe: 24
- Gambia: 25
- Togo: 26
- Equatorial Guinea: 32
- Gabon: 54
- Cameroon: 58

Middle East & North Africa
- Sudan: 8
- Occupied Palestinian Territory: 18

Asia & Pacific
- Nepal: 11
- Cambodia: 16
- Indonesia: 27
- Mongolia: 48
- Viet Nam: 51
- Philippines: 53

CEE/CIS & Baltic States
- Tajikistan: 6
- Azerbaijan: 9
- Albania: 24
- Armenia: 36
- Uzbekistan: 43
- Yugoslavia: 43
- Rep. of Moldova: 56
- Ukraine: 73

Know where to get tested (%)

Sources: UNICEF/MICS, 1999-2001; Measure DHS, 1998-2001.

responsibilities they have to themselves and others as a result. Young women who are pregnant and test HIV positive should be offered special care to safeguard their own health and minimize the risk of passing the virus to their baby.

Because young people are particularly socially and emotionally vulnerable, VCT must be properly sustained, with follow-up provided. Post-test support services, especially for young people who are HIV positive, should serve as a safety net to help them continue to meet their health, psychosocial and financial needs.

VCT services can be integrated into existing services – antenatal care clinics, family health services, youth-friendly clinics – and should be accessible to young people from marginalized groups such as sex workers and migrants. Confidentiality must be respected at all times. VCT services can also be provided through youth clubs, free-standing clinics or mobile vans.

Despite the importance of VCT, in many countries fewer than 50 per cent of young people know where they can be tested for HIV. In Cambodia,

for example, only 16 per cent of girls aged 15 to 19 know where to go for testing; in Zimbabwe only two out of five know where to be tested. Test kits are unavailable in many of the countries most affected by AIDS, which seriously undermines the effectiveness of counselling.

6 Work with young people, promote their participation.

Energetic, enthusiastic and creative, young people are a tremendous resource in all areas of HIV prevention and care. Their input is invaluable in programme design and outreach, ensuring that prevention and care efforts are meaningful to young people, that information is communicated through effective channels, and that the messages conveyed are relevant to their everyday lives.

Involving young people in prevention efforts educates them about HIV and gives them a sense of responsibility and pride. With the right skills, young people can be extremely effective messengers. They are already tapped into their own peer networks and speak the same language as the group they are trying to reach.

Young people are already participating in prevention efforts in many ways. They are starting HIV/AIDS prevention clubs in schools, directing youth-initiated projects in their communities, and working with governments and non-governmental organizations to develop, implement and monitor programmes. The most effective projects are those that are sustained over time, enabling young people to feel challenged and engaged and to assume a lasting sense of responsibility.

True youth participation is a partnership in which both young people and adults have agreed to their responsibilities. Adults need to ensure that young people are continuously informed, trained, motivated and supported in all of their

INCREASED EDUCATION = INCREASED KNOWLEDGE OF WHERE TO GET TESTED

% of young women (aged 12 - 24) who know where to get an HIV test, by level of education – Suriname, 2000

Source: Suriname UNICEF/MICS, 2000.

YOUNG PEOPLE
ALREADY TAKING THE LEAD

- In Ibadan, Nigeria, girl apprentice tailors employed in small workshops were trained as peer educators, returning to their workshops to talk about HIV and the risks of unprotected sex and to brief their peers on how to negotiate condom use. Girls reached by the peer educators were significantly better able to protect themselves from coerced sex than girls who had not received such information.

- In three communities of Lima, Peru, where high unemployment has led to widespread delinquency, 240 young people between the ages of 10 and 24 were trained to educate their peers about a healthy and responsible sex life. They counselled some 5,000 adolescents in person, and reached a further 45,000 by speaking on the radio, singing on public transport and putting on exhibitions at fairs.

- In Nepal, an interactive radio programme, *Chatting with My Best Friend,* is produced and hosted by and for young people, to encourage them to discuss the issues and problems of growing up. The programme offers an avenue to discuss common problems such as boy-girl relationships and communication with parents. Since the launch of the programme, the young hosts have received an average of 100 to 200 letters a week.

- The Mathare Youth Sports Association in Nairobi, Kenya, trains its footballers to be peer educators and role models for HIV/AIDS awareness, prevention and counselling programmes. The members of the senior squad, better known and therefore better able to influence their peers, were the first to be trained. They stress abstinence from sex, but for those who are sexually active, they emphasize the importance of using condoms and staying faithful to one partner.

- In Poland, young people have been trained as 'field counsellors', visiting cafés, youth clubs and other gathering places to educate their peers who are experimenting with drugs on the risks posed by substance abuse, HIV/AIDS and STIs. The young counsellors are trained to assess individual needs and offer appropriate information and referrals.

HIV prevention efforts, according to their ability as this evolves. Young people need to demonstrate commitment and be reliable and active contributors. The most effective partnerships build young people's knowledge, confidence and skills, enabling them to play an increasing role in determining the areas and extent of their involvement and responsibility. The more they learn through experience, the better able they are to take responsibility and turn their concern into action.

Peer education

Serving as peer educators is an effective way for young people to participate in HIV prevention and care efforts. For many young people, their peers serve as a major source of information on sexual issues. Properly trained, peer educators can dispel misconceptions, shatter myths and present information on preventing HIV in a way that other young people will find pertinent.

Peer educators can be trained to provide information, build skills, counsel, or distribute condoms. They can do their work on street corners and in clubs, churches, factories, schools and universities – wherever young people gather and feel comfortable.

Peer educators are very effective in reaching individuals and groups at especially high risk, including males having sex with males, young people who are sexually exploited, gang members, homeless youth and those who use drugs. Many of these young people distrust adults too strongly for adult social workers to reach them. But peer educators are members of the communities they aim to reach; they meet these young people on their own territory, speak the same language and, most importantly, treat them with respect.

Successful peer education programmes require resources and support from their community and commitment from both adults and young people. They also need to be sustained in the long term, since young people require a steady flow of accurate information over time to reinforce their knowledge and maintain positive changes in their behaviour. Since peer educators often receive little or no pay, other forms of incentive, recognition or compensation are needed to keep them actively engaged.

7 Engage young people who are living with HIV/AIDS.

A major challenge in HIV prevention is to convince young people that HIV/AIDS can indeed strike anyone. Among the most effective ways to do this is for young people living with HIV/AIDS to share their own experiences. Young people living with HIV/AIDS are in a strategic position to reinforce information about the need to adopt and maintain safe behaviours. They, more than anyone else, can convey the message that individuals must make every effort to ensure that no one else contracts HIV from them. They can reduce the stigma associated with HIV by showing that the virus can infect anyone. They can be effective role models for how to live healthy, productive lives with HIV. They can make major contributions to the design and implementation of prevention and care efforts.

Unfortunately, in places where stigma and discrimination remain strong, these young people can suffer grievous harm from revealing their HIV status. People living with HIV must be left entirely free to choose whether to 'go public', when and with whom. When they do so, they must receive social support and legal protection allowing them to lead normal lives. All young people living with HIV need medical care to prevent progression of the disease, as well as other support services.

In the San Francisco Bay area in the United States, BAY Positives provides counselling, support groups, case management, education, outreach, retreats, holistic treatment (acupuncture, massage) and social events for young people aged 26 and under living with HIV. This peer-based agency reaches out to young people with HIV of all sexual orientations, those who are recovering from drug and alcohol abuse and those who have been sexually abused and have low self-esteem. One of the major strengths of BAY Positives is the agency's established network of community-based organizations and programmes where young people can be referred for appropriate help. The agency offers career training, health care and education services. The staff members and clients of BAY Positives share similar experiences: all the staff were once members themselves.

8 Create safe and supportive environments.

Providing young people with information and skills without ensuring that they feel safe and supported at home, at school and in their community severely limits their ability to protect themselves from HIV. Parents, schools and social institutions need to be supplied with the knowledge and skills to create an environment in which girls and boys are safe from harm, cared for equally and treated with respect.

Schools and communities must be unequivocal in condemning sexual violence, abuse and exploitation, particularly of children and adolescents. Governments must make sexual violence unacceptable by enacting and enforcing laws that protect young women and men from all forms of sexual violence, inside and outside marriage, as well as imposing criminal penalties on their

abusers. Mass media and educational campaigns must encourage equality between men and women and denounce all forms of violence against women, children and adolescents.

9 Reach out to young people most at risk.

This is an especially difficult challenge, but a vital one, both to protect young people and to prevent concentrated epidemics from spreading into the wider population. The young people at especially high risk for contracting HIV – males having sex with males, children living on the street, child soldiers, young refugees, children orphaned by AIDS, those who use drugs, those who are sexually exploited – are often on the periphery of society and face enormous difficulties in obtaining help.

They need access to livelihoods, education and services to enable them to build their future. Interventions for them must take into account the range of constraints they face and help to establish an environment marked by respect, acceptance and stability. This is key to enabling them to reintegrate into society.

Harm reduction – a treatment approach that seeks to minimize the most harmful consequences of unsafe behaviour – can be especially effective with young people engaged in high-risk behaviours. When applied to drug use, for example, the approach underpins longer-term strategies to end or reduce drug use by taking immediate steps to reduce the chief harms from drug use, including the transmission of HIV/AIDS, by such measures as providing clean needles and condoms.

Children and adolescents orphaned by AIDS require special protection and legislation. Policies and laws on the care of orphans must be developed

---

TARGETED INTERVENTIONS WORK

Decreases in HIV seroprevalence rates among sex workers in Cambodia, 1997-2000

■ Under 20 years old   ■ 20 years or older

Sources: Cambodia HIV sentinel surveillance 2000; Ministry of Health, National Center for HIV/AIDS, Dermatology and STDs; Family Health International (FHI), 2000.

in the best interest of each child, bearing in mind his or her right to be raised in a caring family environment. Legislation must define standards of protection and care for orphans, promote legal fostering and adoption, establish fair inheritance and property rights and expand community-based care, with institutional care considered only as a last resort. Where institutional care is offered, programmes must be developed to integrate children back into their communities at the earliest opportunity.

10 Strengthen partnerships, monitor progress.

Protecting young people from HIV is too big a job for any one sector of society. To make a real and lasting difference, the commitment and resources of all sectors must be mobilized and coordinated, and channelled to families and communities. There must be a commitment to bring people together at every level – community, nation, region, worldwide – to invest in young people. The partners must include non-governmental and civil society organizations, including faith-based organizations and the private sector; governments; young people; academic and research institutions, private foundations; bilateral donor agencies; and the United Nations and other multilateral agencies.

Defeating HIV/AIDS will also require tracking change, both in the infection rates and in the knowledge, awareness and behaviour of young people. Collecting information on their knowledge and behaviour will not only help to monitor progress towards the goals set in June 2001 at the United Nations General Assembly Special Session on HIV/AIDS, it will also help to identify which programmes are succeeding and why.

THE RIGHT TO KNOW

Young people have the right:

- To know about sex and their sexuality

- To know the basic facts on HIV/AIDS and have the necessary life skills to protect themselves from HIV and other STIs

- To know their HIV status

- To know how to protect themselves if they are living with HIV/AIDS

- To know where to get medical, emotional and psychological support if they are living with HIV/AIDS

- To know how to protect their peers and families from HIV

- To know how to protect those in their communities who are living with HIV/AIDS

- To know about and participate in HIV education programmes tailored for youth

- To know their rights and entitlements, and the commitments that governments have made to them

- To know how to protect, claim and realize these rights.

STATISTICAL TABLES

The following two tables contain statistics that help convey the impact of HIV/AIDS on young people worldwide. Epidemiological, behavioural, social, economic, demographic, impact and knowledge indicators are included.

TABLE 1 — HIV/AIDS INDICATORS FOR COUNTRIES, AREAS, TERRITORIES

COUNTRY, AREA OR TERRITORY	DEMOGRAPHICS (2001) Population (thousands) TOTAL	AGE 10-14	AGE 15-24	Young people as a % of total population AGE 10-24	% of population urbanized	GNI per capita (US$) 2000	Type of epidemic (2001)	Est. no. young people with HIV/AIDS Female 15-24 LOW	HIGH	Male 15-24 LOW	HIGH	% young people with HIV/AIDS Female 15-24 LOW	HIGH	Male 15-24 LOW	HIGH	% of adults with HIV/AIDS AGE 15-49
Afghanistan	22,474	2,706	4,343	31	22	250 x	L	-	-	-	-	-	-	-	-	-
Albania	3,145	311	551	27	42	1100	L	-	-	-	-	-	-	-	-	-
Algeria	30,841	3,526	6,690	33	61	1590	L	-	-	-	-	-	-	-	-	0.1*
Andorra	90	-	-	-	93	d	-	-	-	-	-	-	-	-	-	-
Angola	13,527	1,742	2,576	32	35	240	G	54,000	95,000	21,000	37,000	4.1	7.3	1.6	2.8	5.5
Antigua and Barbuda	65	-	-	-	37	9190	-	-	-	-	-	-	-	-	-	-
Argentina	37,488	3,361	6,685	27	90	7440	C	8,900	13,000	23,000	35,000	0.27	0.40	0.69	1.0	0.7
Armenia	3,788	371	704	28	70	520	C	160	240	650	970	0.05	0.07	0.18	0.27	0.2
Australia	19,338	1,336	2,718	21	85	20530	C	160	240	1,300	1,900	0.01	0.02	0.09	0.14	0.1
Austria	8,075	467	941	17	65	25220	C	440	660	860	1,300	0.10	0.14	0.18	0.27	0.2
Azerbaijan	8,096	877	1,514	30	58	610	L	<100	150	340	600	0.01	0.02	0.04	0.08	<0.1
Bahamas	308	29	56	28	89	15010	G	540	1,100	490	1,000	2.0	4.1	1.7	3.6	3.5
Bahrain	652	60	103	25	93	7640 x	L	-	-	-	-	-	-	-	-	0.3
Bangladesh	140,369	16,960	28,680	33	25	380	L	980	1,700	1,100	1,900	0.01	0.01	0.01	0.01	<0.1
Barbados	268	20	42	23	51	9280	G	-	-	-	-	-	-	-	-	1.2*
Belarus	10,147	793	1,606	24	72	2990	C	1,000	2,100	3,100	6,400	0.13	0.26	0.38	0.79	0.3
Belgium	10,264	611	1,232	18	97	24630	C	580	870	580	870	0.10	0.14	0.09	0.14	0.2
Belize	231	28	50	34	55	2940	G	390	590	220	330	1.6	2.4	0.88	1.3	2.0
Benin	6,446	861	1,327	34	43	380	G	20,000	30,000	6,200	9,300	3.0	4.5	0.94	1.4	3.6
Bhutan	2,141	274	423	33	7	550	L	-	-	-	-	-	-	-	-	<0.1
Bolivia	8,516	1,000	1,657	31	63	1000	L	290	600	620	1,300	0.04	0.07	0.07	0.15	0.1
Bosnia and Herzegovina	4,067	305	616	23	44	1260	L	-	-	-	-	-	-	-	-	<0.1*
Botswana	1,554	209	355	36	51	3300	G	53,000	80,000	23,000	34,000	30.0	45.0	12.9	19.3	38.8
Brazil	172,559	16,765	34,158	30	82	3570	C	65,000	98,000	88,000	130,000	0.38	0.58	0.51	0.77	0.7
Brunei Darussalam	335	35	58	28	73	24630 x	L	-	-	-	-	-	-	-	-	-
Bulgaria	7,867	497	1,140	21	70	1510	L	-	-	-	-	-	-	-	-	<0.1*
Burkina Faso	11,856	1,617	2,478	35	19	230	G	98,000	150,000	39,000	58,000	7.8	11.7	3.2	4.8	6.5
Burundi	6,502	933	1,367	35	9	110	G	55,000	97,000	24,000	43,000	8.0	14.1	3.6	6.3	8.3
Cambodia	13,441	1,758	2,643	33	16	260	G	26,000	39,000	10,000	15,000	2.0	3.0	0.77	1.2	2.7
Cameroon	15,203	1,965	3,167	34	50	570	G	160,000	240,000	69,000	100,000	10.1	15.2	4.3	6.5	11.8
Canada	31,015	2,067	4,132	20	77	21050	C	2,800	4,200	4,600	6,900	0.14	0.21	0.22	0.33	0.3
Cape Verde	437	52	94	33	63	1330	-	-	-	-	-	-	-	-	-	-
Central African Republic	3,782	472	755	32	42	290	G	42,000	62,000	17,000	26,000	10.8	16.2	4.7	7.0	12.9
Chad	8,135	1,018	1,555	32	24	200	G	22,000	45,000	12,000	25,000	2.8	5.8	1.5	3.2	3.6
Chile	15,402	1,442	2,507	26	86	4600	C	1,000	2,100	3,000	6,100	0.08	0.17	0.23	0.48	0.3
China	1,284,972	116,776	200,371	25	33	840	C	60,000	110,000	120,000	210,000	0.06	0.11	0.11	0.20	0.1
Colombia	42,803	4,403	8,083	29	74	2080	C	4,800	10,000	23,000	47,000	0.12	0.25	0.55	1.2	0.4
Comoros	727	90	156	34	34	380	L	-	-	-	-	-	-	-	-	-
Congo	3,110	390	595	32	63	630	G	15,000	32,000	6,300	13,000	5.1	10.5	2.1	4.4	7.2
Congo, Democratic Republic of	52,522	6,887	9,985	32	31	100 x	G	210,000	380,000	110,000	190,000	4.3	7.5	2.1	3.7	4.9
Cook Islands	20	-	-	-	60	-	-	-	-	-	-	-	-	-	-	-
Costa Rica	4,112	436	790	30	48	3960	C	670	1,400	1,500	3,200	0.18	0.36	0.38	0.79	0.6
Côte d'Ivoire	16,349	2,162	3,572	35	47	660	G	120,000	180,000	42,000	63,000	6.7	10.0	2.3	3.5	9.7
Croatia	4,655	294	639	20	58	4510	L	-	-	-	-	-	-	-	-	<0.1
Cuba	11,237	867	1,496	21	76	1170 x	L	200	410	450	930	0.03	0.06	0.06	0.12	<0.1
Cyprus	790	65	123	24	57	11950 x	L	-	-	-	-	-	-	-	-	0.3
Czech Republic	10,260	641	1,518	21	75	4920	L	-	-	-	-	-	-	-	-	<0.1
Denmark	5,333	311	589	17	85	32020	C	150	230	330	490	0.05	0.08	0.11	0.16	0.2
Djibouti	644	81	127	32	84	840	G	-	-	-	-	-	-	-	-	-
Dominica	71	-	-	-	71	3260	-	-	-	-	-	-	-	-	-	-
Dominican Republic	8,507	936	1,697	31	66	2100	G	18,000	27,000	15,000	22,000	2.2	3.3	1.7	2.5	2.5
East Timor	750	118	148	36	8	-	- s	-	-	-	-	-	-	-	-	-
Ecuador	12,880	1,388	2,603	31	66	1210	C	1,300	2,600	2,600	5,400	0.10	0.20	0.20	0.41	0.3
Egypt	69,080	8,156	14,246	32	46	1490	L	-	-	-	-	-	-	-	-	<0.1

38

COUNTRY, AREA OR TERRITORY	EDUCATION				Have heard of AIDS (%)	KNOWLEDGE (1998-2001)								SEXUAL BEHAVIOUR (1998-2001)			
	Net primary school attendance/enrolment (%) (1995-2001)		Secondary school enrolment ratio (1995-2001) (gross)			% who know that a person can protect themselves from HIV infection by:			% who know HIV can't be transmitted by:		% who know healthy-looking people can be infected with HIV		Have sufficient knowledge to protect themselves (%)	Median age at first sex		% sexually active by age 15	
	FEMALE	MALE	FEMALE	MALE	FEMALE 15-24	One faithful uninfected partner FEMALE 15-24	Consistent condom use FEMALE 15-24	Abstaining from sex FEMALE 15-19	Supernatural means FEMALE 15-24	Mosquito bites FEMALE 15-24	FEMALE 15-24	MALE 15-24	FEMALE 15-24	FEMALE 20-24	MALE 20-24	FEMALE 20-24	MALE 20-24
Afghanistan	11 s	36 s	11	32	-	-	-	-	-	-	-	-	-	-	-	-	-
Albania	90 s	90 s	38	37	93	55	42	37	-	14	40	-	4	-	-	-	-
Algeria	96 s	98 s	62	65	-	-	-	-	-	-	-	-	-	-	-	-	-
Andorra	-	-	-	-	-	-	-	-	-	-	-	-	-	-	-	-	-
Angola	48 s	52 s	-	-	-	-	-	-	-	-	-	-	-	-	-	-	-
Antigua and Barbuda	-	-	-	-	-	-	-	-	-	-	-	-	-	-	-	-	-
Argentina	96	96	81	73	-	-	-	-	-	-	-	-	-	-	-	-	-
Armenia	-	-	91 x	85 x	93	48	42	-	-	-	53	-	-	19.7y	-	1	-
Australia	95	95	155	150	91 y	-	-	-	-	-	-	-	-	-	-	-	-
Austria	91	90	102	105	-	-	-	-	-	-	-	-	-	-	-	-	-
Azerbaijan	88 s	88 s	81	73	61	14	11	8	15	7	35	-	-	-	-	-	-
Bahamas	99	99	91 x	88 x	-	-	-	-	-	-	-	-	-	-	-	-	-
Bahrain	98	96	98	91	-	-	-	-	-	-	-	-	-	-	-	-	-
Bangladesh	83 s	81 s	13 x	25 x	33	-	-	-	-	-	22	29	-	-	-	-	-
Barbados	100	100	80 x	90 x	-	-	-	-	-	-	-	-	-	-	-	-	-
Belarus	84	87	95	91	-	-	-	-	-	-	-	-	-	-	-	-	-
Belgium	98	96	151	142	-	-	-	-	-	-	-	-	-	18.7x	18.1x	9 x	15 x
Belize	90	92	52 x	47 x	-	-	-	-	-	-	-	-	-	-	-	-	-
Benin	50	75	10	24	95	-	-	-	-	-	41 x	66	-	17.2x	17.6x	15 x	19 x
Bhutan	47	58	2 x	7 x	-	-	-	-	-	-	-	-	-	-	-	-	-
Bolivia	87 s	88 s	34 x	40 x	78	63	57	50	62	40	55	74	-	19.6	17.1y	6	21
Bosnia and Herzegovina	95 s	94 s	-	-	97	55	53	41	-	-	74	-	-	-	-	-	-
Botswana	85 s	83 s	68	61	95	76	76	79	70	47	79	-	-	17.4x	-	-	-
Brazil	95 s	95 s	36 x	31 x	99	-	-	-	-	-	79 x	80	-	18.7x	16.7y, x	10 x	34 x
Brunei Darussalam	91	90	82	71	-	-	-	-	-	-	-	-	-	-	-	-	-
Bulgaria	98	98	76	77	-	-	-	-	-	-	-	-	-	18.7	-	-	-
Burkina Faso	22 s	32 s	6 x	11 x	84	-	-	-	-	-	42	64	-	17.3	20.0	10	8
Burundi	44 s	49 s	5	9	85	71	47	62	68	48	66	-	24	20.4x	-	2 x	-
Cambodia	65 s	66 s	18	30	94	64	64	55	60	52	62	-	37	21.9	-	3	-
Cameroon	71 s	75 s	22 x	32 x	90	51	46	42	48	34	54	63	16	16.3	17.0	26	16
Canada	94	96	105	105	-	-	-	-	-	-	-	-	-	17.8x	-	-	-
Cape Verde	97	100	56	54	99	-	-	-	-	-	53	60	-	-	-	26	45
Central African Republic	39 s	47 s	6 x	15 x	65	49	20	39	27	22	46	-	5	16.0x	-	28 x	16 x
Chad	33 s	46 s	4	15	70	32	21	26	28	13	28	-	5	16.0x	18.4x	33 x	7 x
Chile	89	90	78	72	-	97	74	-	-	67	-	-	-	18.6	17.4	-	-
China	99	99	65	72	74 y	-	-	-	-	-	-	-	-	-	-	-	-
Colombia	90 s	90 s	75	70	98	-	-	-	-	-	84	-	-	18.4	-	9	-
Comoros	55	65	16 x	21 x	87	42	41	30	41	27	55	-	10	20.9x	18.1x	10 x	17 x
Congo	-	-	45	62	-	-	-	-	-	-	-	-	-	-	-	12	25
Congo, Democratic Republic of	51	66	19 x	32 x	-	-	-	-	-	-	-	-	-	-	-	-	-
Cook Islands	97	99	-	-	-	-	-	-	-	-	-	-	-	-	-	-	-
Costa Rica	91	92	50	47	-	-	-	-	-	-	-	-	-	-	-	-	-
Côte d'Ivoire	52	61 s	16	33	93	55	53	48	45	38	51	-	16	16.2	17.5	24	18
Croatia	96	93	83	81	-	-	-	-	-	-	-	-	-	-	-	-	-
Cuba	95	93	85	76	100	88	89	55	91	65	91	-	-	-	-	-	-
Cyprus	96	96	99	96	-	-	-	-	-	-	-	-	-	-	-	-	-
Czech Republic	91	92	100	97	-	-	-	-	-	-	-	-	-	-	-	-	-
Denmark	99	99	122	120	-	-	-	-	-	-	-	-	-	17.0	17.5x	32 x	27 x
Djibouti	28	39	12	17	-	-	-	-	-	-	-	-	-	-	-	-	-
Dominica	89	89	-	-	-	-	-	-	-	-	-	-	-	-	-	-	-
Dominican Republic	94 s	94 s	47 x	34 x	99	87	73	73	87	47	89	92	33	18.7x	-	13 x	26 x
East Timor	-	-	-	-	17 y	-	-	-	-	-	-	-	-	-	-	-	-
Ecuador	90 s	90 s	55 x	53 x	89	-	-	-	-	55	59	-	-	19.3	-	8	-
Egypt	84 s	88 s	70	80	66 y	-	-	-	-	-	-	-	-	-	-	-	-

TABLE 1   HIV/AIDS INDICATORS FOR COUNTRIES, AREAS, TERRITORIES

COUNTRY, AREA OR TERRITORY	Population (thousands) TOTAL	AGE 10-14	AGE 15-24	Young people as a % of total population AGE 10-24	% of population urbanized	GNI per capita (US$) 2000	Type of epidemic (2001)	Estimated no. Female 15-24 LOW	HIGH	Male 15-24 LOW	HIGH	% Female 15-24 LOW	HIGH	Male 15-24 LOW	HIGH	% of adults AGE 15-49
El Salvador	6,400	696	1,333	32	47	1990	C	1,500	3,200	3,400	7,000	0.23	0.48	0.50	1.0	0.6
Equatorial Guinea	470	57	86	30	49	1170 x	G	780	1,600	390	810	1.8	3.7	0.91	1.9	3.4
Eritrea	3,816	480	736	32	19	170	G	11,000	20,000	7,400	13,000	3.1	5.5	2.0	3.5	2.8
Estonia	1,377	103	207	23	69	3410	C	460	800	1,900	3,300	0.45	0.79	1.8	3.2	1.0
Ethiopia	64,459	8,203	12,380	32	18	100	G	350,000	620,000	200,000	350,000	5.6	10.0	3.2	5.6	6.4
Fiji	823	85	167	31	50	1830	L	-	-	-	-	-	-	-	-	<0.1
Finland	5,178	318	660	19	68	24900	L	<100	<100	<100	150	0.02	0.03	0.03	0.04	<0.1
France	59,453	3,806	7,714	19	76	23670	C	5,400	8,100	8,200	12,000	0.14	0.21	0.21	0.31	0.3
Gabon	1,262	142	217	28	82	3180	G	-	-	-	-	-	-	-	-	-
Gambia	1,337	151	240	29	33	330	G	1,100	2,200	410	850	0.88	1.8	0.34	0.71	1.6
Georgia	5,239	412	822	24	61	590	L	<100	100	200	410	0.01	0.03	0.05	0.10	<0.1
Germany	82,007	4,679	9,151	17	88	25050	C	1,600	2,400	3,700	5,500	0.04	0.05	0.08	0.12	0.1
Ghana	19,734	2,476	4,250	34	39	350	G	44,000	82,000	20,000	37,000	2.1	3.9	0.95	1.8	3.0
Greece	10,623	559	1,433	19	60	11960	C	360	540	780	1,200	0.05	0.08	0.11	0.16	0.2
Grenada	94	-	-	-	38	3520	-	-	-	-	-	-	-	-	-	-
Guatemala	11,687	1,494	2,436	34	40	1690	G	6,600	14,000	7,300	15,000	0.55	1.1	0.59	1.2	1.0
Guinea	8,274	1,002	1,669	32	34	450	G	-	-	-	-	-	-	-	-	-
Guinea-Bissau	1,227	147	230	31	24	180	G	2,200	4,600	780	1,600	1.9	4.0	0.69	1.4	2.8
Guyana	763	73	160	31	39	770	G	2,100	4,300	1,700	3,600	2.6	5.4	2.1	4.4	2.7
Haiti	8,270	1,112	1,824	36	36	510	G	29,000	61,000	24,000	50,000	3.2	6.7	2.6	5.5	6.1
Holy See	1	-	-	-	100	-	-	-	-	-	-	-	-	-	-	-
Honduras	6,575	830	1,373	34	54	850	G	8,100	12,000	6,700	10,000	1.2	1.8	0.96	1.4	1.6
Hungary	9,917	609	1,421	20	64	4740	L	100	180	490	860	0.01	0.03	0.07	0.12	0.1
Iceland	281	22	42	23	93	31090	C	-	-	-	-	-	-	-	-	0.2
India	1,025,096	109,177	193,619	30	29	460	G,C,L	430,000	890,000	220,000	470,000	0.46	0.96	0.22	0.46	0.8
Indonesia	214,840	21,738	42,501	30	42	570	C	9,500	14,000	11,000	17,000	0.05	0.07	0.05	0.08	0.1
Iran	71,369	9,708	16,110	36	62	1630	L	550	1,100	2,200	4,600	0.01	0.01	0.03	0.06	<0.1
Iraq	23,584	2,976	4,760	33	77	2170 x	L	-	-	-	-	-	-	-	-	<0.1
Ireland	3,841	286	685	25	59	22960	L	130	200	170	260	0.04	0.06	0.05	0.07	0.1
Israel	6,172	543	1,046	26	91	16310 x	C	-	-	-	-	-	-	-	-	0.1
Italy	57,503	2,803	6,471	16	67	20010	C	6,600	9,900	7,500	11,000	0.21	0.31	0.23	0.34	0.4
Jamaica	2,598	272	522	31	57	2440	G	1,800	2,700	1,700	2,600	0.69	1.0	0.66	0.98	1.2
Japan	127,335	6,392	15,642	17	79	34210	C	2,000	3,000	1,200	1,700	0.03	0.04	0.01	0.02	<0.1
Jordan	5,051	584	1,045	32	75	1680	L	-	-	-	-	-	-	-	-	<0.1
Kazakhstan	16,095	1,630	2,979	29	57	1190	L	360	650	1,400	2,500	0.02	0.04	0.09	0.17	0.1
Kenya	31,293	4,349	7,197	37	34	360	G	450,000	670,000	170,000	260,000	12.4	18.7	4.8	7.2	15.0
Kiribati	84	-	-	-	40	950	-	-	-	-	-	-	-	-	-	-
Korea, Democratic People's Republic of	22,428	1,946	3,416	24	61	a	L	-	-	-	-	-	-	-	-	-
Korea, Republic of	47,069	3,230	7,572	23	82	8910	L	290	440	660	980	0.01	0.01	0.02	0.03	<0.1
Kuwait	1,971	265	479	38	98	19020 x	L	-	-	-	-	-	-	-	-	-
Kyrgyzstan	4,986	586	977	31	33	270	L	-	-	-	-	-	-	-	-	<0.1
Lao People's Democratic Republic	5,403	690	1,057	32	24	290	L	<100	170	180	330	0.02	0.03	0.03	0.06	<0.1
Latvia	2,406	182	352	22	69	2860	C	340	500	1,300	2,000	0.19	0.29	0.75	1.1	0.4
Lebanon	3,556	378	663	29	90	3750	L	-	-	-	-	-	-	-	-	-
Lesotho	2,057	245	410	32	29	540	G	50,000	100,000	23,000	49,000	24.8	51.4	11.3	23.5	31.0
Liberia	3,108	350	759	36	46	490 x	G	-	-	-	-	-	-	-	-	-
Libyan Arab Jamahiriya	5,408	590	1,279	35	88	5540 x	L	-	-	-	-	-	-	-	-	0.2
Liechtenstein	33	-	-	-	23	d	-	-	-	-	-	-	-	-	-	-
Lithuania	3,689	285	537	22	69	2900	L	-	-	-	-	0.03	0.06	0.10	0.22	0.1
Luxembourg	442	26	54	18	92	44340	L	-	-	-	-	-	-	-	-	0.2
Madagascar	16,437	2,013	3,161	31	30	260	L	3,000	4,500	860	1,300	0.19	0.28	0.05	0.08	0.3
Malawi	11,572	1,505	2,331	33	26	170	G	140,000	210,000	60,000	90,000	11.9	17.9	5.1	7.6	15.0
Malaysia	22,633	2,322	4,267	29	58	3380	C	1,900	2,900	12,000	18,000	0.09	0.14	0.56	0.84	0.4
Maldives	300	40	62	34	26	1460	L	-	-	-	-	-	-	-	-	0.1
Mali	11,677	1,461	2,287	32	31	240	G	15,000	32,000	10,000	21,000	1.4	2.8	0.89	1.8	1.7

COUNTRY, AREA OR TERRITORY	Net primary school attendance/enrolment (%) (1995-2001) FEMALE	MALE	Secondary school enrolment ratio (1995-2001) (gross) FEMALE	MALE	Have heard of AIDS (%) FEMALE 15-24	One faithful uninfected partner FEMALE 15-24	Consistent condom use FEMALE 15-24	Abstaining from sex FEMALE 15-19	Supernatural means FEMALE 15-24	Mosquito bites FEMALE 15-24	% who know healthy-looking people can be infected with HIV FEMALE 15-24	MALE 15-24	Have sufficient knowledge to protect themselves (%) FEMALE 15-24	Median age at first sex FEMALE 20-24	MALE 20-24	% sexually active by age 15 FEMALE 20-24	MALE 20-24
El Salvador	78	78	35	30	88	-	-	-	-	58 t	69 t	-	-	18.7	-	10	-
Equatorial Guinea	89	89	-	-	76	29	26	23	31	15	46	-	4	-	-	-	-
Eritrea	35	40	17	24	80	-	-	-	-	-	54 x	67 x	-	17.9 x	-	16 x	-
Estonia	86	87	108	100	-	-	-	-	-	-	-	-	-	18.4 x	-	-	-
Ethiopia	37	51	10	14	82	62	37	-	-	-	39	54	-	18.1	21.3 y	19	3
Fiji	100	99	65 x	64 x	-	-	-	-	-	-	-	-	-	-	-	-	-
Finland	98	98	125	110	-	-	-	-	-	-	-	-	-	18.0 x	18.0 x	18 x	20 x
France	100	100	111	112	-	-	-	-	-	-	-	-	-	18.4 x	17.9 x	2 x	6 x
Gabon	83	82	-	-	98	65	79	59	-	-	72	81	-	16.2	15.7	24	36
Gambia	49 s	54 s	19	30	84	56	52	41	48	31	53	-	15	-	-	-	-
Georgia	98 s	98 s	76	78	90	21 t	24 t	-	-	39	47	-	-	-	-	2	-
Germany	87	86	103	105	-	-	-	-	-	-	-	-	-	-	-	-	-
Ghana	74 s	75 s	29 x	45 x	97	74	70	73	-	-	71	77	22 y	17.5	19.5	10	8
Greece	90	90	96	95	-	-	-	-	-	-	-	-	-	19.0 x	17.5 x	5 x	5 x
Grenada	97	98	-	-	-	-	-	-	-	-	-	-	-	-	-	-	-
Guatemala	75 s	80 s	24	26	90 t	19 t	43 t	-	-	42 t	41 t	-	-	19.0	-	11	-
Guinea	30	49	7	20	96	-	-	-	-	-	60	56	-	16.0	17.5	32	21
Guinea-Bissau	39 s	46 s	4 x	9 x	61	26	32	18	28	27	31	-	8	-	-	-	-
Guyana	92	97	78	73	96	73	69	58	77	57	84	-	-	-	-	-	-
Haiti	43	42	20 x	21 x	97	55	46	-	18	28	68	78	14	18.2	16.7 y	14	34
Holy See	-	-	-	-	-	-	-	-	-	-	-	-	-	-	-	-	-
Honduras	86	85	37 x	29 x	98	-	-	-	-	61 x	78 x	85 x	-	18.4 x	15.7 x	10 x	33 x
Hungary	96	97	99	96	-	-	-	-	-	-	-	-	-	18.5 x	18.0 x	-	-
Iceland	98	98	108	109	-	-	-	-	-	-	-	-	-	16.9 x	16.8 x	22 x	38 x
India	73 s	79 s	39	59	37	57 t	59 t	71 t	-	-	~26	-	-	18.0	21.0	-	-
Indonesia	93	93	48	55	69	40	23	-	47	32	32	-	-	20.4 x	-	6 x	-
Iran	96	99	73	81	-	-	-	-	-	-	-	-	-	-	-	-	-
Iraq	88	98	32	51	-	-	-	-	-	-	-	-	-	-	-	-	-
Ireland	100	100	122	113	-	-	-	-	-	-	-	-	-	-	-	-	-
Israel	-	-	89 x	84 x	-	-	-	-	-	-	-	-	-	-	-	-	-
Italy	100	100	95	94	-	-	-	-	-	48 y,x	-	-	-	22.0 x	19.0 x	-	2
Jamaica	94	92	67 x	63 x	99 y	-	-	-	-	-	-	-	-	17.1 x	-	14 x	-
Japan	100	100	100 x	99 x	-	-	-	-	-	-	-	-	-	-	-	-	-
Jordan	94	95	54 x	52 x	99	-	-	-	-	-	57 x	-	-	-	-	-	-
Kazakhstan	100	100	89	80	96	38	39	12	-	-	63	66	-	20.0	18.6	2	5
Kenya	75 s	73 s	22	26	90	75	52	67	76	55	75	80	26	17.3	16.2	17	34
Kiribati	-	-	-	-	-	-	-	-	-	-	-	-	-	-	-	-	-
Korea, Democratic People's Republic of	-	-	-	-	-	-	-	-	-	-	-	-	-	-	-	-	-
Korea, Republic of	98	97	102	102	81 y	-	-	-	-	-	-	-	-	-	-	-	-
Kuwait	85	89	65	65	-	-	-	-	-	-	-	-	-	-	-	-	-
Kyrgyzstan	97	98	83	75	-	-	-	-	-	-	-	-	-	19.5 x	-	0.3 x	-
Lao People's Democratic Republic	67 s	71 s	23	34	59 y	-	-	-	-	-	-	-	-	-	-	-	-
Latvia	92	88	85	82	-	-	-	-	-	-	-	-	-	18.5 x	18.2 x	-	-
Lebanon	98 s	98 s	85	78	-	-	-	-	-	-	-	-	-	-	-	-	-
Lesotho	68 s	62 s	36	25	81	50	58	38	56	36	46	-	18	-	-	5 x	10 x
Liberia	31	43	12 x	31 x	63 y	44 t	49 t	19 t	-	-	-	-	-	15.5	17.4	39	16
Libyan Arab Jamahiriya	-	-	95 x	95 x	-	-	-	-	-	-	-	-	-	-	-	-	-
Liechtenstein	-	-	-	-	-	-	-	-	-	-	-	-	-	-	-	-	-
Lithuania	-	-	88	85	-	-	-	-	-	-	-	-	-	19.5 x	18.6 x	-	-
Luxembourg	-	-	76 x	72 x	-	-	-	-	-	-	-	-	-	-	-	-	-
Madagascar	58 s	57 s	16	16	59	38	33	28	-	12	27	-	5	17.0 x	-	19 x	-
Malawi	83 s	83 s	12	21	99	75	66	71	-	69	84	89	34	17.1	17.7	18	20
Malaysia	94 s	94 s	66	58	83 y	-	-	-	-	-	-	-	-	-	-	-	-
Maldives	97	99	49 x	49 x	99 t	-	-	-	-	-	-	-	-	-	-	-	-
Mali	33	47	7	14	81	-	-	-	-	-	37 x	47 x	-	15.9 x	18.7 x	25 x	7 x

COUNTRY, AREA OR TERRITORY	Population (thousands) TOTAL	AGE 10-14	AGE 15-24	Young people as a % of total population AGE 10-24	% of population urbanized	GNI per capita (US$) 2000	Type of epidemic (2001)	Estimated no. Female 15-24 LOW	HIGH	Male 15-24 LOW	HIGH	% Female 15-24 LOW	HIGH	Male 15-24 LOW	HIGH	% of adults AGE 15-49
Malta	392	28	59	22	91	9410 x	L	-	-	-	-	-	-	-	-	0.1
Marshall Islands	52	-	-	-	72	1970	-	-	-	-	-	-	-	-	-	-
Mauritania	2,747	333	539	32	59	370	C	-	-	-	-	-	-	-	-	-
Mauritius	1,171	97	209	26	42	3800	L	-	-	-	-	-	-	-	-	0.1
Mexico	100,368	10,673	19,934	30	75	5080	C	6,500	11,000	26,000	47,000	0.06	0.12	0.26	0.47	0.3
Micronesia (Federated States of)	126	-	-	-	29	2110	-	-	-	-	-	-	-	-	-	-
Moldova, Republic of	4,285	399	775	27	46	400	C	330	680	1,200	2,400	0.09	0.18	0.30	0.62	0.2
Monaco	34	-	-	-	100	d	-	-	-	-	-	-	-	-	-	-
Mongolia	2,559	325	548	34	64	390	L	-	-	-	-	-	-	-	-	<0.1
Morocco	30,430	3,352	6,239	32	57	1180	L	-	-	-	-	-	-	-	-	0.1
Mozambique	18,644	2,299	3,688	32	41	210	G	200,000	350,000	81,000	140,000	10.6	18.8	4.4	7.8	13.0
Myanmar	48,364	5,084	9,582	30	28	220 x	G	-	-	-	-	-	-	-	-	-
Namibia	1,788	234	355	33	31	2050	G	34,000	51,000	16,000	24,000	19.4	29.1	8.9	13.3	22.5
Nauru	13	-	-	-	100	-	-	-	-	-	-	-	-	-	-	-
Nepal	23,593	2,817	4,524	31	12	220	C	4,000	8,300	4,100	8,500	0.18	0.38	0.17	0.36	0.5
Netherlands	15,930	980	1,845	18	90	25140	C	660	990	1,500	2,300	0.07	0.11	0.16	0.24	0.2
New Zealand	3,808	295	518	21	86	13080	L	<100	<100	110	170	0.01	0.02	0.04	0.06	0.1
Nicaragua	5,208	643	1,115	34	57	420	C	270	570	830	1,700	0.05	0.10	0.15	0.31	0.2
Niger	11,227	1,444	2,180	32	21	180	G	-	-	-	-	-	-	-	-	-
Nigeria	116,929	15,073	23,713	33	45	260	G	540,000	820,000	290,000	430,000	4.7	7.0	2.4	3.6	5.8
Niue	2	-	-	-	33	-	-	-	-	-	-	-	-	-	-	-
Norway	4,488	293	533	18	76	33650	L	<100	120	160	240	0.03	0.05	0.06	0.09	0.1
Occupied Palestinian Territory	3,311	429	621	32	95	1610	-	-	-	-	-	-	-	-	-	-
Oman	2,622	352	516	33	85	4940 x	L	-	-	-	-	-	-	-	-	0.1
Pakistan	144,971	17,718	28,082	32	38	470	L	4,600	9,500	5,800	12,000	0.03	0.07	0.04	0.08	0.1
Palau	20	-	-	-	73	c	-	-	-	-	-	-	-	-	-	-
Panama	2,899	293	531	28	57	3260	G	2,300	4,200	3,600	6,500	0.90	1.6	1.4	2.4	1.5
Papua New Guinea	4,920	561	1,006	32	18	760	C	1,200	2,400	1,200	2,400	0.25	0.53	0.21	0.45	0.7
Paraguay	5,636	682	1,120	32	57	1450	C	-	-	-	930	-	-	-	0.16	-
Peru	26,093	2,828	5,299	31	73	2100	C	3,500	6,200	7,900	14,000	0.13	0.23	0.30	0.53	0.4
Philippines	77,131	9,087	15,669	32	59	1040	L	880	1,300	820	1,200	0.01	0.02	0.01	0.02	<0.1
Poland	38,577	2,830	6,568	24	66	4200	C	870	1,800	1,900	4,000	0.03	0.06	0.06	0.12	0.1*
Portugal	10,033	546	1,407	19	66	11060	C	1,000	1,500	2,300	3,500	0.15	0.22	0.33	0.49	0.5
Qatar	575	48	73	21	93	12000 x	L	-	-	-	-	-	-	-	-	-
Romania	22,388	1,667	3,574	23	57	1670	L	-	-	-	-	-	-	-	-	<0.1
Russian Federation	144,664	11,203	23,087	24	78	1660	C	60,000	91,000	170,000	260,000	0.53	0.79	1.5	2.2	0.9
Rwanda	7,949	1,030	1,772	35	6	230	G	80,000	120,000	35,000	52,000	9.0	13.4	3.9	5.9	8.9
Saint Kitts and Nevis	38	-	-	-	34	6660	-	-	-	-	-	-	-	-	-	-
Saint Lucia	149	14	31	30	38	4070	-	-	-	-	-	-	-	-	-	-
Saint Vincent and Grenadines	114	-	-	-	56	2690	-	-	-	-	-	-	-	-	-	-
Samoa	159	22	36	36	22	1460	-	-	-	-	-	-	-	-	-	-
San Marino	27	-	-	-	89	d	-	-	-	-	-	-	-	-	-	-
Sao Tome and Principe	140	-	-	-	47	290	-	-	-	-	-	-	-	-	-	-
Saudi Arabia	21,028	2,703	4,090	32	86	6900 x	L	-	-	-	-	-	-	-	-	-
Senegal	9,662	1,232	1,934	33	48	500	G	4,100	6,200	1,400	2,200	0.43	0.65	0.15	0.22	0.5
Seychelles	81	-	-	-	65	7310	-	-	-	-	-	-	-	-	-	-
Sierra Leone	4,587	548	877	31	37	130	G	22,000	45,000	7,000	15,000	4.9	10.2	1.6	3.4	7.0
Singapore	4,108	289	508	19	100	24740	L	300	450	300	460	0.12	0.19	0.12	0.17	0.2
Slovakia	5,403	398	912	24	58	3700	L	-	-	-	-	-	-	-	-	<0.1
Slovenia	1,985	119	287	20	51	10070	L	-	-	-	-	-	-	-	-	<0.1
Solomon Islands	463	57	92	32	20	630	-	-	-	-	-	-	-	-	-	-
Somalia	9,157	1,147	1,765	32	28	120 x	G	-	-	-	-	-	-	-	-	1.0

COUNTRY, AREA OR TERRITORY	EDUCATION				KNOWLEDGE (1998-2001)									SEXUAL BEHAVIOUR (1998-2001)			
	Net primary school attendance/enrolment (%) (1995-2001)		Secondary school enrolment ratio (1995-2001) (gross)		Have heard of AIDS (%)	% who know that a person can protect themselves from HIV infection by:			% who know HIV can't be transmitted by:		% who know healthy-looking people can be infected with HIV		Have sufficient knowledge to protect themselves (%)	Median age at first sex		% sexually active by age 15	
						One faithful uninfected partner	Consistent condom use	Abstaining from sex	Supernatural means	Mosquito bites							
	FEMALE	MALE	FEMALE	MALE	FEMALE 15-24	FEMALE 15-24	FEMALE 15-24	FEMALE 15-19	FEMALE 15-24	FEMALE 15-24	FEMALE 15-24	MALE 15-24	FEMALE 15-24	FEMALE 20-24	MALE 20-24	FEMALE 20-24	MALE 20-24
Malta	100	100	82	86	-	-	-	-	-	-	-	-	-	-	-	-	-
Marshall Islands	-	-	-	-	-	-	-	-	-	-	-	-	-	-	-	-	-
Mauritania	53 s	55 s	11	21	76	28	17	21	-	-	30	39	-	-	-	-	-
Mauritius	98	97	66	63	-	-	-	-	-	-	-	-	-	-	-	-	-
Mexico	97 s	97 s	64	64	-	-	-	-	-	-	-	-	-	20.7 x	-	-	-
Micronesia (Federated States of)	-	-	-	-	-	-	-	-	-	-	-	-	-	-	-	-	-
Moldova, Republic of	99 s	98 s	81	78	96	63	56	29	72	38	79	-	-	-	-	5 x	-
Monaco	-	-	-	-	-	-	-	-	-	-	-	-	-	-	-	-	-
Mongolia	92 s	91 s	65	48	93	79	77	43	74	58	57	-	-	-	-	-	-
Morocco	64	77	34	44	-	-	-	-	-	-	-	-	-	-	-	-	-
Mozambique	40	47	5	9	83	-	-	-	-	-	38 x	59 x	-	16.0 x	18.5y, x	32 x	13 x
Myanmar	69 s	68 s	30 x	29 x	90 y	-	-	-	-	-	-	-	-	-	-	-	-
Namibia	88	84	66	56	98	77	86	-	-	-	-	-	-	18.7 x	-	6 x	-
Nauru	97	99	-	-	-	-	-	-	-	-	-	-	-	-	-	-	-
Nepal	60 s	71 s	25 x	49 x	45	-	-	-	-	-	29	-	-	17.3 x	-	18 x	-
Netherlands	100	100	129	134	-	-	-	-	-	-	-	-	-	18.3 x	18.3x	12 x	17 x
New Zealand	100	100	116	110	-	-	-	-	-	-	-	-	-	17.2 x	-	-	-
Nicaragua	80	80	53	45	95	-	-	-	-	-	75	80	-	18.1	15.8	14	35
Niger	31 s	44 s	5	9	72	43	30	37	34	19	22	43	5	15.7	20.3y	36	4
Nigeria	54 s	58 s	28 x	33 x	75	-	-	-	-	-	45	51	-	18.1	19.6	21	11
Niue	100	100	-	-	-	-	-	-	-	-	-	-	-	-	-	-	-
Norway	100	100	116	121	-	-	-	-	-	-	-	-	-	18.0 x	19.0x	10 x	6 x
Occupied Palestinian Territory	94 s	93 s	-	-	92	54	38	-	-	30	49	-	-	-	-	-	-
Oman	88	90	65	68	-	-	-	-	-	-	-	-	-	-	-	-	-
Pakistan	41 s	50 s	17 x	33 x	-	-	-	-	-	-	-	-	-	-	-	-	-
Palau	-	-	-	-	-	-	-	-	-	-	-	-	-	-	-	-	-
Panama	91	91	65 x	60 x	-	-	-	-	-	-	-	-	-	-	-	-	-
Papua New Guinea	-	-	11	17	66 x	-	-	-	-	-	45 x	-	-	-	-	-	-
Paraguay	80 s	92 s	45	42	-	-	-	-	-	-	78	-	-	17.9 x	-	7 x	-
Peru	87 s	87 s	67	72	88	34	34	-	-	-	72	-	-	19.6	-	7	19
Philippines	91 s	88 s	75 x	71 x	91	70	54	-	-	37	67	-	4	-	-	2	-
Poland	-	-	97	98	-	-	-	-	-	-	-	-	-	19.6 x	19.7x	-	-
Portugal	100	100	111 x	102 x	-	-	-	-	-	-	-	-	-	20.0 x	17.0x	-	7
Qatar	92	96	79	81	-	-	-	-	-	-	-	-	-	-	-	-	-
Romania	96	96	78	79	99	82	92	-	-	70	70	76	-	19.5	17.3	3	19
Russian Federation	93	93	91 x	83 x	-	-	-	-	-	-	~84 x	-	-	-	-	8 x	-
Rwanda	66 s	65 s	9 x	12 x	99	72	63	79	-	60	64	69	23	20.3 y	20.6y	4	7
Saint Kitts and Nevis	86	92	-	-	-	-	-	-	-	-	-	-	-	-	-	-	-
Saint Lucia	-	-	-	-	-	-	-	-	-	-	-	-	-	-	-	-	-
Saint Vincent and Grenadines	78	90	-	-	-	-	-	-	-	-	-	-	-	-	-	-	-
Samoa	91	94	66	59	-	-	-	-	-	-	-	-	-	-	-	-	-
San Marino	-	-	-	-	-	-	-	-	-	-	-	-	-	-	-	-	-
Sao Tome and Principe	-	-	-	-	95	25	32	20	47	37	65	-	11	-	-	-	-
Saudi Arabia	73	81	57	65	-	-	-	-	-	-	-	-	-	-	-	-	-
Senegal	45 s	54 s	12	20	70	50	38	33	45	24	36	66	10	18.8 x	-	13 x	7 x
Seychelles	100	100	-	-	-	-	-	-	-	-	-	-	-	-	-	-	-
Sierra Leone	40 s	43 s	13 x	22 x	59	32	30	30	37	29	35	-	16	-	-	-	-
Singapore	92	93	77	70	89 y	-	-	-	-	-	-	-	-	-	-	-	-
Slovakia	-	-	96	92	-	-	-	-	-	-	-	-	-	-	-	-	-
Slovenia	94	95	93	90	-	-	-	-	-	-	-	-	-	18.0 x	17.0x	-	-
Solomon Islands	-	-	14 x	21 x	-	-	-	-	-	-	-	-	-	-	-	-	-
Somalia	11 s	13 s	6 x	10 x	28	8	2	6	6	3	11	-	1	-	-	-	-

	DEMOGRAPHICS (2001)							EPIDEMIOLOGY								
	Population (thousands)			Young people as a % of total population	% of population urbanized	GNI per capita (US$) 2000	Type of epi-demic (2001)	Estimated no. of young people living with HIV/AIDS, end-2001				% of young people living with HIV/AIDS, end-2001				% of adults living with HIV/AIDS, end-2001
								Female 15-24		Male 15-24		Female 15-24		Male 15-24		
COUNTRY, AREA OR TERRITORY	TOTAL	AGE 10-14	AGE 15-24	AGE 10-24				LOW	HIGH	LOW	HIGH	LOW	HIGH	LOW	HIGH	AGE 15-49
South Africa	43,792	4,776	9,031	32	51	3020	G	930,000	1,400,000	380,000	580,000	20.5	30.8	8.5	12.8	20.1
Spain	39,921	2,045	5,542	19	78	14960	C	5,200	7,800	12,000	17,000	0.19	0.29	0.41	0.62	0.5
Sri Lanka	19,104	1,722	3,655	28	24	870	L	490	740	400	590	0.03	0.04	0.02	0.03	<0.1
Sudan	31,809	3,689	6,254	31	37	320	G	63,000	130,000	22,000	46,000	2.0	4.2	0.70	1.5	2.6
Suriname	419	44	90	32	75	1350 x	G	440	910	360	750	0.99	2.1	0.79	1.6	1.2
Swaziland	938	120	193	33	27	1290	G	31,000	46,000	12,000	18,000	31.6	47.4	12.2	18.3	33.4
Sweden	8,833	586	1,016	18	83	26780	L	180	260	270	410	0.04	0.05	0.05	0.08	0.1
Switzerland	7,170	416	779	17	68	38120	C	1,200	1,800	1,500	2,200	0.32	0.47	0.37	0.55	0.5
Syrian Arab Republic	16,610	2,258	3,735	36	55	990	L	-	-	-	-	-	-	-	-	-
Tajikistan	6,135	827	1,245	34	28	170	L	-	-	-	-	-	-	-	-	<0.1
Tanzania, United Republic of	35,965	4,712	7,449	34	34	280	G	240,000	360,000	110,000	160,000	6.4	9.7	2.8	4.3	7.8
The former Yugoslav Republic of Macedonia	2,044	160	334	24	62	1710	L	-	-	-	-	-	-	-	-	<0.1
Thailand	63,584	5,488	11,682	27	22	2010	G	77,000	120,000	51,000	78,000	1.3	2.0	0.88	1.3	1.8
Togo	4,657	593	948	33	34	300	G	22,000	34,000	7,800	12,000	4.7	7.1	1.6	2.5	6.0
Tonga	99	-	-	-	39	1660	-	-	-	-	-	-	-	-	-	-
Trinidad and Tobago	1,300	125	271	30	75	4980	G	2,800	5,900	2,100	4,500	2.1	4.4	1.6	3.3	2.5
Tunisia	9,562	1,018	2,019	32	66	2090	L	-	-	-	-	-	-	-	-	-
Turkey	67,632	5,925	13,368	29	76	3090	L	-	-	-	-	-	-	-	-	<0.1*
Turkmenistan	4,835	591	949	32	45	840	L	-	-	-	-	-	-	-	-	<0.1
Tuvalu	10	-	-	-	53	-	-	-	-	-	-	-	-	-	-	-
Uganda	24,023	3,163	4,838	33	15	310	G	90,000	130,000	38,000	58,000	3.7	5.6	1.6	2.4	5.0
Ukraine	49,112	3,614	7,390	22	68	700	C	23,000	41,000	53,000	94,000	0.63	1.1	1.4	2.5	1.0
United Arab Emirates	2,654	256	420	25	86	18060 x	L	-	-	-	-	-	-	-	-	-
United Kingdom	59,542	3,912	7,224	19	90	24500	C	1,500	2,200	3,000	4,500	0.04	0.06	0.08	0.12	0.1
United States	285,926	20,773	38,980	21	77	34260	C	34,000	51,000	76,000	110,000	0.18	0.27	0.38	0.57	0.6
Uruguay	3,361	269	524	24	92	6090	C	410	620	1,100	1,700	0.16	0.24	0.42	0.63	0.3
Uzbekistan	25,257	3,191	5,155	33	37	610	L	<100	<100	160	330	<0.01	<0.01	0.01	0.01	<0.1
Vanuatu	202	26	40	32	20	1140	-	-	-	-	-	-	-	-	-	-
Venezuela	24,632	2,703	4,802	30	87	4310	C	-	-	-	18,000	-	-	-	0.74	0.5*
Viet Nam	79,175	9,290	16,137	32	20	390	C	11,000	16,000	20,000	31,000	0.13	0.20	0.25	0.38	0.3
Yemen	19,114	2,366	3,427	30	25	380	L	-	-	-	-	-	-	-	-	0.1
Yugoslavia	10,538	760	1,612	23	53	b	L	-	-	-	-	-	-	-	-	0.2
Zambia	10,649	1,399	2,215	34	40	300	G	180,000	280,000	72,000	110,000	16.8	25.2	6.5	9.7	21.5
Zimbabwe	12,852	1,776	2,840	36	36	480	G	370,000	560,000	140,000	210,000	26.4	39.6	9.9	14.9	33.7
REGIONAL AVERAGES								FEMALE 15-24		MALE 15-24		FEMALE 15-24		MALE 15-24		
Sub-Saharan Africa	633,830	80,956	128,479	33	35	528		5,700,000		2,800,000		8.9		4.4		
East and Southern Africa	319,094	40,523	65,022	33	30	683		4,100,000		2,000,000		12.7		6.3		
West and Central Africa	314,736	40,434	63,457	33	39	342		1,600,000		780,000		5.1		2.5		
Middle East and North Africa	350,660	42,861	73,018	33	58	1326		110,000		46,000		0.3		0.1		
South Asia	1,378,049	151,414	263,388	30	29	455		670,000		390,000		0.5		0.3		
East Asia and Pacific	1,893,781	178,926	317,498	26	36	1125		340,000		400,000		0.2		0.2		
Latin America and Caribbean	521,051	53,428	101,190	30	76	3713		240,000		320,000		0.5		0.6		
CEE/CIS and Baltic States	476,604	39,463	80,550	25	67	2038		85,000		340,000		0.2		0.8		
Industrialized countries	865,073	54,219	110,697	19	79	28077		83,000		160,000		0.2		0.3		
Developing countries	4,925,609	522,537	912,332	29	40	1175		7,100,000		4,000,000		1.6		0.9		
Least developed countries	684,615	84,868	135,900	32	27	290		2,800,000		1,400,000		4.1		2.1		
World	6,119,050	601,266	1,074,821	27	47	5192		7,300,000		4,500,000		1.4		0.8		

COUNTRY, AREA OR TERRITORY	EDUCATION				KNOWLEDGE (1998-2001)									SEXUAL BEHAVIOUR (1998-2001)			
	Net primary school attendance/enrolment (%) (1995-2001)		Secondary school enrolment ratio (1995-2001) (gross)		Have heard of AIDS (%)	% who know that a person can protect themselves from HIV infection by:			% who know HIV can't be transmitted by:		% who know healthy-looking people can be infected with HIV		Have sufficient knowledge to protect themselves (%)	Median age at first sex		% sexually active by age 15	
						One faithful uninfected partner	Consistent condom use	Abstaining from sex	Supernatural means	Mosquito bites							
	FEMALE	MALE	FEMALE	MALE	FEMALE 15-24	FEMALE 15-24	FEMALE 15-24	FEMALE 15-19	FEMALE 15-24	FEMALE 15-24	FEMALE 15-24	MALE 15-24	FEMALE 15-24	FEMALE 20-24	MALE 20-24	FEMALE 20-24	MALE 20-24
South Africa	86	88	91	76	96 y	88 t	87 t	78	-	46 t	54	-	-	17.8	-	7	-
Spain	100	100	128	116	-	-	-	-	-	-	-	-	-	20.1x	18.7x	-	-
Sri Lanka	-	-	78	71	-	-	-	-	-	-	-	-	-	-	-	-	-
Sudan	37	43	19	21	43	24	12	-	19	18	16	-	2	-	-	-	-
Suriname	91 s	88 s	58 x	50 x	94	58	58	42	57	46	70	-	27	-	-	-	-
Swaziland	100	100	54	55	97	61	63	63	75	55	81	-	27	-	-	-	-
Sweden	100	100	153	128	-	-	-	-	-	-	-	-	-	17.1x	-	-	-
Switzerland	96	96	88 x	94 x	-	-	-	-	-	-	-	-	-	18.6x	18.3x	-	-
Syrian Arab Republic	98 s	99 s	40	45	-	-	-	-	-	-	-	-	-	-	-	-	-
Tajikistan	93 s	93 s	72	81	13	6	5	3	6	4	8	-	~3	-	-	-	-
Tanzania, United Republic of	55 s	51 s	5	6	96	64	62	62	-	54	65	68	26	17.4	17.5	17	14
The former Yugoslav Republic of Macedonia	96	97	62	64	-	-	-	-	-	-	-	-	-	-	-	-	-
Thailand	79	82	37 x	38 x	91 y	-	-	-	-	-	-	-	-	-	19.0x	0 x	2 x
Togo	64 s	74 s	14	40	96	74	63	55	53	48	67	73	20	16.5	18.0	18	12
Tonga	93	98	-	-	-	-	-	-	-	-	-	-	-	-	-	-	-
Trinidad and Tobago	88	88	75	72	97	82	54	63	87	71	95	-	33	15.0	14.0	-	-
Tunisia	93 s	95 s	63	66	-	-	-	-	-	-	-	-	-	-	-	-	-
Turkey	70 s	74 s	48	68	86	-	-	-	-	-	62	69	-	-	-	-	-
Turkmenistan	80 s	81 s	-	-	64	29	21	21	-	-	42	-	-	21.6 t	-	0	-
Tuvalu	100	100	-	-	-	-	-	-	-	-	-	-	-	-	-	-	-
Uganda	83	92	9	15	100 t	83	68	-	-	47	76	83	28	16.7	19.4y	21	8
Ukraine	-	-	94 x	88 x	100	61	57	21	61	39	78	-	-	17.8	-	23	-
United Arab Emirates	98	98	82	77	-	-	-	-	-	-	-	-	-	-	-	-	-
United Kingdom	98	97	139	120	-	-	-	-	-	-	-	-	-	17.4x	17.1x	16 x	25 x
United States	95	94	97	98	-	-	-	-	-	-	-	-	-	17.2x	-	-	-
Uruguay	93	92	92	77	-	-	-	-	-	-	-	-	-	-	-	-	-
Uzbekistan	78 s	78 s	87 x	99 x	64	32	22	17	22	15	41	-	-	19.7x	-	0.4 x	-
Vanuatu	-	-	18 x	23 x	-	-	-	-	-	-	-	-	-	-	-	-	-
Venezuela	85	83	46	33	-	-	-	-	-	-	-	-	-	-	-	-	-
Viet Nam	93 s	94 s	41 x	44 x	85	63	60	34	71	44	63	-	-	-	-	-	-
Yemen	40 s	75 s	14	53	-	-	-	-	-	-	-	-	-	-	-	-	-
Yugoslavia	97 s	98 s	66	62	92	58	63	25	-	43	65	-	-	-	-	-	-
Zambia	68 s	67 s	21 x	34 x	95	78	59	79	68	63	75	84	26	16.6x	16.0x	22 x	32 x
Zimbabwe	86 s	84 s	44	52	96	73	73	-	-	-	74	83	17 y	18.9	19.5	5	8
REGIONAL AVERAGES																	
Sub-Saharan Africa	57	63	22	28													
East and Southern Africa	63	67	25	26													
West and Central Africa	51	59	20	30													
Middle East and North Africa	77	84	55	64													
South Asia	68	74	33	52													
East Asia and Pacific	95	95	60	66													
Latin America and Caribbean	91	92	53	49													
CEE/CIS and Baltic States	85	86	82	82													
Industrialized countries	96	96	107	105													
Developing countries	78	82	46	55													
Least developed countries	55	62	14	23													
World	80	83	54	61													

NOTES:

a: Range $750 or less.

b: Range $756 to $2995.

c: Range $2996 to $9265.

d: Range $9266 or more.

s: Attendance data derived from household survey.

t: Adults (15-49).

x: Indicates data that refer to years other than those specified in the column heading, differ from the standard definition or refer to only part of a country.

y: Data is for young people, but age range differs from standard.

*: Older estimate, not enough data were available to produce an estimate of HIV prevalence for end-2001.

~: Approximately.

TABLE 1

Demographics

Population 2001: total; aged 10-14; aged 15-24

Young people as a % of total population, aged 10-24

% of population urbanized: % of total population living in urban areas according to the national definition used in the most recent population census.

Source: United Nations Population Division.

GNI per capita (US$) 2000: Gross national income is the sum value added by all resident producers plus any product taxes (less subsidies) not included in the valuation of output plus net receipts of primary income (compensation of employees and property income) from abroad. GNI per capita is gross national income divided by mid-year population. GNI per capita in US dollars, as of the year 2000, is converted using the *World Bank Atlas* method.

Source: World Bank.

Epidemiology

Type of epidemic (2001): The level of the HIV epidemic (low, concentrated or generalized). **L:** Low HIV prevalence, which does not consistently exceed 5% in any sub-population whose behaviour places them at highest risk (those attending sexually transmitted infection clinics; injecting drug users; sex workers; and men who have sex with men). **C:** Concentrated HIV prevalence, which has been consistently over 5% in at least one sub-population at highest risk, and is below 1% in the general adult population (aged 15-49 years) in urban areas. **G:** Generalized HIV prevalence, which has reached 1% in the general adult population (aged 15-49 years).

Source: Walker, N., et al., 'Epidemiological analysis of the quality of HIV sero-surveillance in the world: How well do we track the epidemic?' AIDS 2001, 15:1545-1554; and more recent country-specific updates.

Estimated no. of young people living with HIV/AIDS: aged 15-24 years living with HIV/AIDS at the end of 2001.

Sources: UNAIDS; UNICEF; WHO.

% of young people (aged 15-24 years) living with HIV/AIDS: The estimated number of young people living with HIV/AIDS at the end of 2001 divided by the 2001 total number of young people aged 15-24.

Sources: UNAIDS; UNICEF; WHO.

% of adults living with HIV/AIDS, end-2001, aged 15-49: The estimated number of adults aged 15-49 living with HIV/AIDS at the end of 2001, divided by the 2001 adult population.

Education

Net primary school attendance/enrolment (%) (1995-2001): The number of children attending or enrolled in primary school who belong to the age group that officially corresponds to primary schooling, divided by the total population of the same age group. The data is derived from national household surveys that asked children of primary school age questions about their school attendance. Where this information was not available, the indicator was derived from administrative school data collected by national Ministries of Education together with primary-school-age population data (enrolment).

Sources: Multiple Indicator Cluster Surveys (MICS), UNICEF; Demographic and Health Surveys (DHS), Macro International; UNESCO.

Gross secondary school enrolment ratio: The number of children enrolled in secondary school, regardless of age, divided by the population of the age group that officially corresponds to the secondary school level.

Source: UNESCO.

Knowledge about transmission of HIV

Have heard of AIDS: % of young women (aged 15-24 years) who report having heard of AIDS. The value for young women is presented since young women usually have lower knowledge levels about HIV/AIDS than young men and in generalized epidemics higher HIV prevalence rates are found in young women.

Sources: MICS, UNICEF; DHS, Macro International; Centers for Disease Control and Prevention (CDC); other national surveys.

% who know that people can protect themselves from HIV infection by: % of young people who know the three primary methods of protection: (1) having sex with one faithful, uninfected partner; (2) consistent condom use; and (3) abstaining from sex. The third option, abstinence, an extremely important prevention option for young people, is only reported for the age group 15-19 because it is less of a prevention option for the older age group (20-24 years) where the majority are already sexually active.

Sources: MICS, UNICEF; DHS, Macro International; CDC; other national surveys.

% who know HIV can't be transmitted by: % of young people who correctly reject the two most common misconceptions about HIV/AIDS transmission or prevention, and who know that a healthy-looking person can be infected with HIV.

Sources: MICS, UNICEF; DHS, Macro International; CDC; other national surveys.

Have sufficient knowledge to protect themselves: % of all young people (aged 15-24 years) who both correctly identify ways of preventing the sexual transmission of HIV and who reject major misconceptions about HIV transmission or prevention. This indicator is a composite of two prevention methods (condom use and one faithful partner) and three misconceptions.

Sources: MICS, UNICEF, DHS, Macro International.

Sexual behaviour

Median age at first sex: The age by which one half of young men and women aged 20-24 have had penetrative sex (median age), of all young people (aged 20-24 years) surveyed.

Sources: DHS, Macro International; CDC; other national surveys.

% sexually active by age 15: % of young men and women (aged 20-24 years) who report having had first penetrative sex before their 15th birthday.

Sources: DHS, Macro International; CDC; other national surveys.

TABLE 2

HIV prevalence among pregnant women

HIV prevalence among pregnant women (aged 15-24): % of blood samples taken from pregnant women aged 15-24 that test positive for HIV during 'unlinked anonymous sentinel surveillance' at selected antenatal clinics. The data is presented separately for young women aged 15-19 and 20-24 years attending antenatal care clinics in 'major urban areas' and 'outside major urban areas'. For each of the groups, the table gives the year of the most recent surveillance round, the number of surveillance sites and the median value. An [n] following a year denotes a nationwide number, [u] urban, [r] rural.

Sources: Country Sentinel Surveillance Reports (1997-2002) and HIV/AIDS Surveillance Database; US Census Bureau; International Programs Center; Health Studies Branch, 2002.

Access

Antenatal care coverage: % of women aged 15-19 and 20-24 years who were attended at least once during pregnancy by skilled health personnel (doctors, nurses or midwives).

Sources: MICS, UNICEF; DHS, Macro International; CDC; other national surveys.

% who know a source of condoms: % of young men and women aged 15-24.

Sources: MICS, UNICEF; DHS, Macro International; CDC; other national surveys.

Risky sexual behaviour

% of never-married young people having sex in past 12 months: Young people aged 15-24.

Sources: DHS, Macro International; CDC, MICS, UNICEF and other national surveys.

% who used condom at last high-risk sex in past 12 months: % of young men and women (aged 15-24) who say they used a condom the last time they had sex with a non-marital, non-cohabiting partner, of those who have had sex with such a partner in the last 12 months.

Sources: DHS, Macro International; CDC; MICS, UNICEF and other national surveys.

HIV testing

Know a place to get tested: % of young women (aged 15-24) who know where to get an HIV test.

Sources: MICS, UNICEF; DHS, Macro International.

Have been tested: % of young women (aged 15-24) who have been tested for HIV.

Sources: MICS, UNICEF; DHS, Macro International.

Informed about result of test: % of young women who have been tested for HIV and informed of the result.

Sources: MICS, UNICEF; DHS, Macro International.

Impact

Orphan school attendance rate as a % of non-orphan attendance rate (1995-2001): % of children aged 10-14 in a household survey who lost both natural parents and who are currently attending school as a % of non-orphaned children of the same age who live with at least one parent and who are attending school.

Sources: MICS, UNICEF; DHS, Macro International.

Estimated no. of primary school children who lost a teacher to HIV/AIDS (end-1999): The number of children is based on the estimated number of teachers who died due to AIDS in 1999, multiplied by the student-teacher ratio.

Sources: UNAIDS; UNICEF.

COUNTRY	HIV PREVALENCE AMONG PREGNANT WOMEN (AGED 15-24) Major urban areas YEAR [# SITES]	MEDIAN 15-19	MEDIAN 20-24	Outside major urban areas YEAR [# SITES]	MEDIAN 15-19	MEDIAN 20-24	ACCESS Antenatal care coverage (%) 1995-2001 AGE <20	AGE 20-24	% who know a source of condoms (1998-2001*) FEMALE 15-24	MALE 15-24	RISKY SEXUAL BEHAVIOUR (1998-2001) % of never-married young people having sex in past 12 months FEMALE 15-24	MALE 15-24	% who used condom at last high-risk sex in past 12 months FEMALE 15-24	MALE 15-24	HIV TESTING (1998-2001) (%) Know a place to get tested FEMALE 15-24	Have been tested FEMALE 15-24	Informed about result of test FEMALE 15-24	IMPACT Orphan school attendance rate as a % of non-orphan attendance rate (1995-2001)	No. of primary school children who lost a teacher to HIV/AIDS (end-1999)
Angola	-	-	-	-	-	-	66	71	-	-	-	-	-	-	-	-	-	-	3,300
Bahamas	-	-	-	-	-	-	-	-	-	-	-	-	-	-	-	-	-	-	-
Barbados	-	-	-	-	-	-	-	-	-	-	-	-	-	-	-	-	-	-	-
Belize	-	-	-	-	-	-	-	-	-	-	-	-	-	-	-	-	-	-	-
Benin	1999 [n]	2.2	4.8	1999 [n]	2.2	4.8	83	83	20 x	62 k	-	-	-	-	-	-	-	37	1,800
Botswana	2001 [3]	27.1	34.9	2001 [19]	26.6	46.9	-	-	-	-	-	-	-	-	48	15	-	99	14,000
Burkina Faso	1998 [1]	6.2	8.8	-	-	-	62	64	27	-	24	34	41	55	-	-	-	-	7,400
Burundi	1998 [1]	8.8	15.4	1998 [1]	24	14.3	77	79	-	-	-	-	-	-	28	2	69	69	9,500
Cambodia	2000 [n]	1.9	2.8	2000 [n]	1.9	2.8	45g	39g	33	-	0.2	-	41	-	16	2	-	71	-
Cameroon	2000 [5]	9.5	11.2	2000 [22]	9.3	14.1	74	73	-	-	52	58	16	31	58	-	-	92	19,000
Central African Republic	-	-	-	-	-	-	71	64	-	-	-	-	-	-	24	8	78	89	5,700
Chad	-	-	-	-	-	-	47	42	6 x	-	16 x	36 x	3 x	2 x	9	1	68	93	2,600
Congo	2000 [u]	11	-	-	-	-	-	-	-	-	-	-	-	-	-	-	-	-	3,900
Congo, Democratic Republic of	-	-	-	-	-	-	-	-	-	-	-	-	-	-	-	-	-	-	27,000
Côte d'Ivoire	1998 [3]	4.7	12.2	1997 [9]	7.5	12.1	85	90	68	-	56	61	25	56	19	6	58	77	23,000
Djibouti	-	-	-	-	-	-	-	-	-	-	-	-	-	-	-	-	-	-	500
Dominican Republic	1999 [n]	1.8 (15-24)		1999 [n]	1.8 (15-24)		97	98	74 x	92 x	8 x	52 x	12 x	48 x	8	40	92	87	-
Equatorial Guinea	-	-	-	-	-	-	86	89	-	-	-	-	-	-	32	10	68	-	<100
Eritrea	-	-	-	-	-	-	46g, x	50g, x	14 x	79 k	-	10 x	-	~2 x	-	-	-	-	-
Estonia	-	-	-	-	-	-	-	-	-	-	-	-	-	-	-	-	-	-	-
Ethiopia	2000 [4]	8.9	17.6	2000 [3]	0	4.3	29	27	3	-	8	17	17	30	-	-	-	60	51,000
Gabon	1995 [3]	7.1	2 (20-29)	-	-	-	83g	80g	62N	92N	64	76	33	48	54	14	-	98	960
Gambia	-	-	-	-	-	-	90	93	-	-	-	-	-	-	25	5	81	-	350
Ghana	2000 [5]	1.9	3	2000 [17]	0	1.6	90	87	69	87	30 x	48 x	48 x	57 x	-	-	-	95	11,000
Guatemala	-	-	-	-	-	-	56	64	34 x	-	-	-	-	-	6	27	-	98	-
Guinea	1995 [1]	0.5	2	-	-	-	74	72	19	71	25	49	18	32	-	-	-	115	1,300
Guinea-Bissau	-	-	-	1997 [7]	2.6	8.6	71	70	-	-	-	-	-	-	20	5	84	104	-
Guyana	1997 [1]	3	7	-	-	-	-	-	-	-	-	-	-	-	68	13	84	-	-
Haiti	2000 [n]	3.7	3.8	2000 [n]	3.7	3.8	71 x	72 x	68N	-	21	47	19	30	22	3	-	82	-
Honduras	-	-	-	-	-	-	-	-	-	-	-	-	-	-	-	-	-	-	-
Jamaica	1997 [3]	1.3	1.4	-	-	-	-	-	-	-	-	-	-	-	-	-	-	-	-
Kenya	1997 [1]	12.5	16.2	-	-	-	91	92	56	81	32	56	14	43	58	8	75	75	95,000
Lesotho	1999 [n]	25	41	1999 [n]	25	41	87	90	-	-	-	-	-	-	5	9	69	89	6,200
Liberia	-	-	-	-	-	-	85g	85g	-	-	-	-	-	-	-	-	-	-	-
Malawi	2001 [3]	13.6	25.7	2001 [16]	10.2	20.3	93 x	92 x	76	88	27	49	32	38	72	9	-	92	52,000
Mali	1997 [u]	3.5 (13-24)		-	-	-	49	48	18 x	-	-	37 x	-	-	-	-	-	72	2,000
Mozambique	2000 [2]	13	14.7	2000 [18]	6.3	13.7	70	70	15 x	30 x	61 x	43 x	-	-	-	-	-	35	20,000
Myanmar	2000 [n]	2.9	2.8	2000 [n]	2.9	2.8	-	-	-	-	-	-	-	-	-	-	-	-	-
Namibia	2000 [n]	11.9	20.3	2000 [n]	11.9	20.3	85 x	87 x	-	-	-	-	-	-	-	17	90	-	9,500
Niger	-	-	-	-	-	-	38	41	12	-	8	21	~2	~2	12	0.4	69	69	820
Nigeria	2000 [n]	3	5.8	2000 [n]	3	5.8	47	64	28	-	28	31	-	-	-	-	-	88	85,000
Panama	-	-	-	-	-	-	-	-	-	-	-	-	-	-	-	-	-	-	-
Rwanda	1999 [4]	8.4	12.8	1999 [6]	4.2	7.6	94 x	96 x	35N	74N	4	9	23	55	4	5	-	93	15,000
Sierra Leone	-	-	-	-	-	-	70	76	-	-	-	-	-	-	9	2	38	74	1,900
Somalia	-	-	-	-	-	-	-	-	-	-	-	-	-	-	-	1	17	-	-
South Africa	2000 [n]	16.1	29.1	2000 [n]	16.1	29.1	95g	94g	-	-	55	-	20	-	-	-	-	-	100,000
Sudan	-	-	-	-	-	-	69g, x	73g, x	-	-	-	-	-	-	8	1	58	-	-
Suriname	-	-	-	-	-	-	59	70	-	-	-	-	-	-	59	7	75	89	-
Swaziland	2000 [u]	22	42.2	2000 [3]	30.1	42.5	85	90	-	-	-	-	-	-	5	14	69	86	3,600
Tanzania, United Republic of	2000 [3]	13.2 (15-24)		2000 [9]	16.3 (15-24)		92	95	55	76	39	57	21	31	46	5	-	72	49,000
Thailand	-	-	-	-	-	-	-	-	-	-	-	-	-	-	-	-	-	-	-
Togo	-	-	-	-	-	-	86	87	46	75	53	46	22	41	26	3	70	92	7,300
Trinidad and Tobago	-	-	-	-	-	-	44	75	-	-	-	-	-	-	73	12	76	-	-
Uganda	2000 [2]	7	10.5	2000 [3]	2	11	93	93	57	-	27	31	44	62	36	9	91	94	81,000
Ukraine	1999 [u]	-	0.4	-	-	-	91g	90g	-	-	-	-	-	-	73	57	53	-	-
Zambia	1998 [4]	16.7	26.8	1998 [18]	6	17.5	95	96	72 x	85 x	36 x	57 x	20 x	39 x	57	4	79	88	56,000
Zimbabwe	2000 [u]	27.1	34.8	2000 [r]	28.4	35.3	90	95	62	77	15	34	42	69	40	10	-	85	86,000

Note: Countries with [n], [u] & [r] are not median values but averages for all tested women combined from different sites. The averages are not necessarily weighted in all countries.

g: (20-34) years age group.

N: knows source and could get condom if wanted.

k: (20-24) years age group.

x: Indicates data that refer to years other than those specified in the column heading, differ from the standard definition or refer to only part of a country.

~: Approximately.

LIST OF COUNTRIES, AREAS AND TERRITORIES

Regional averages given at the end of each table are calculated using data from the countries, areas and territories as grouped below.

Sub-Saharan Africa

Angola; Benin; Botswana; Burkina Faso; Burundi; Cameroon; Cape Verde; Central African Republic; Chad; Comoros; Congo; Congo, Democratic Republic of; Côte d'Ivoire; Equatorial Guinea; Eritrea; Ethiopia; Gabon; Gambia; Ghana; Guinea; Guinea-Bissau; Kenya; Lesotho; Liberia; Madagascar; Malawi; Mali; Mauritania; Mauritius; Mozambique; Namibia; Niger; Nigeria; Rwanda; Sao Tome and Principe; Senegal; Seychelles; Sierra Leone; Somalia; South Africa; Swaziland; Tanzania, United Republic of; Togo; Uganda; Zambia; Zimbabwe

Middle East and North Africa

Algeria; Bahrain; Cyprus; Djibouti; Egypt; Iran; Iraq; Jordan; Kuwait; Lebanon; Libyan Arab Jamahiriya; Morocco; Occupied Palestinian Territory; Oman; Qatar; Saudi Arabia; Sudan; Syrian Arab Republic; Tunisia; United Arab Emirates; Yemen

South Asia

Afghanistan; Bangladesh; Bhutan; India; Maldives; Nepal; Pakistan; Sri Lanka

East Asia and Pacific

Brunei Darussalam; Cambodia; China; Cook Islands; East Timor; Fiji; Indonesia; Kiribati; Korea, Democratic People's Republic of; Korea, Republic of; Lao People's Democratic Republic; Malaysia; Marshall Islands; Micronesia, Federated States of; Mongolia; Myanmar; Nauru; Niue; Palau; Papua New Guinea; Philippines; Samoa; Singapore; Solomon Islands; Thailand; Tonga; Tuvalu; Vanuatu; Viet Nam

Latin America and Caribbean

Antigua and Barbuda; Argentina; Bahamas; Barbados; Belize; Bolivia; Brazil; Chile; Colombia; Costa Rica; Cuba; Dominica; Dominican Republic; Ecuador; El Salvador; Grenada; Guatemala; Guyana; Haiti; Honduras; Jamaica; Mexico; Nicaragua; Panama; Paraguay; Peru; Saint Kitts and Nevis; Saint Lucia; Saint Vincent and the Grenadines; Suriname; Trinidad and Tobago; Uruguay; Venezuela

CEE/CIS and Baltic States

Albania; Armenia; Azerbaijan; Belarus; Bosnia and Herzegovina; Bulgaria; Croatia; Czech Republic; Estonia; Georgia; Hungary; Kazakhstan; Kyrgyzstan; Latvia; Lithuania; Moldova, Republic of; Poland; Romania; Russian Federation; Slovakia; Tajikistan; the former Yugoslav Republic of Macedonia; Turkey; Turkmenistan; Ukraine; Uzbekistan; Yugoslavia

Industrialized countries

Andorra; Australia; Austria; Belgium; Canada; Denmark; Finland; France; Germany; Greece; Holy See; Iceland; Ireland; Israel; Italy; Japan; Liechtenstein; Luxembourg; Malta; Monaco; Netherlands; New Zealand; Norway; Portugal; San Marino; Slovenia; Spain; Sweden; Switzerland; United Kingdom; United States

Developing countries

Afghanistan; Algeria; Angola; Antigua and Barbuda; Argentina; Armenia; Azerbaijan; Bahamas; Bahrain; Bangladesh; Barbados; Belize; Benin; Bhutan; Bolivia; Botswana; Brazil; Brunei Darussalam; Burkina Faso; Burundi; Cambodia; Cameroon; Cape Verde; Central African Republic; Chad; Chile; China; Colombia; Comoros; Congo; Congo, Democratic Republic of; Cook Islands; Costa Rica; Côte d'Ivoire; Cuba; Cyprus; Djibouti; Dominica; Dominican Republic; East Timor; Ecuador; Egypt; El Salvador; Equatorial Guinea; Eritrea; Ethiopia; Fiji; Gabon; Gambia; Georgia; Ghana; Grenada; Guatemala; Guinea; Guinea-Bissau; Guyana; Haiti; Honduras; India; Indonesia; Iran; Iraq; Israel; Jamaica; Jordan; Kazakhstan; Kenya; Kiribati; Korea, Democratic People's Republic of; Korea, Republic of; Kuwait; Kyrgyzstan; Lao People's Democratic Republic; Lebanon; Lesotho; Liberia; Libyan Arab Jamahiriya; Madagascar; Malawi; Malaysia; Maldives; Mali; Marshall Islands; Mauritania; Mauritius; Mexico; Micronesia, Federated States of; Mongolia; Morocco; Mozambique; Myanmar; Namibia; Nauru; Nepal; Nicaragua; Niger; Nigeria; Niue; Occupied Palestinian Territory; Oman; Pakistan; Palau; Panama; Papua New Guinea; Paraguay; Peru; Philippines; Qatar; Rwanda; Saint Kitts and Nevis; Saint Lucia; Saint Vincent and the Grenadines; Samoa; Sao Tome and Principe; Saudi Arabia; Senegal; Seychelles; Sierra Leone; Singapore; Solomon Islands; Somalia; South Africa; Sri Lanka; Sudan; Suriname; Swaziland; Syrian Arab Republic; Tajikistan; Tanzania, United Republic of; Thailand; Togo; Tonga; Trinidad and Tobago; Tunisia; Turkey; Turkmenistan; Tuvalu; Uganda; United Arab Emirates; Uruguay; Uzbekistan; Vanuatu; Venezuela; Viet Nam; Yemen; Zambia; Zimbabwe

Least developed countries

Afghanistan; Angola; Bangladesh; Benin; Bhutan; Burkina Faso; Burundi; Cambodia; Cape Verde; Central African Republic; Chad; Comoros; Congo, Democratic Republic of; Djibouti; Equatorial Guinea; Eritrea; Ethiopia; Gambia; Guinea; Guinea-Bissau; Haiti; Kiribati; Lao People's Democratic Republic; Lesotho; Liberia; Madagascar; Malawi; Maldives; Mali; Mauritania; Mozambique; Myanmar; Nepal; Niger; Rwanda; Samoa; Sao Tome and Principe; Senegal; Sierra Leone; Solomon Islands; Somalia; Sudan; Tanzania, United Republic of; Togo; Tuvalu; Uganda; Vanuatu; Yemen; Zambia